W9-AQG-864

LIFE & DEATH DECISIONS

Help in Making Tough Choices About Bioethical Issues

ROBERT D. ORR, M.D.
DAVID L. SCHIEDERMAYER, M.D.
DAVID B. BIEBEL, D. MIN.

NAVPRESS
A MINISTRY OF THE NAVIGATORS
P.O. BOX 6000, COLORADO SPRINGS, COLORADO 80934

© 1990 by Robert D. Orr, David B. Biebel,
    and David L. Schiedermayer
All rights reserved, including translation
Library of Congress Catalog Card Number:
    90-61789
ISBN 08910-92951

The illustrations in this book could all be true, since many of them are based on our clinical or pastoral experiences. The rest are true-to-life possibilities. When based on actual cases, an effort has been made to protect individual privacy. Any remaining resemblance to specific individuals is either by permission or coincidence.

Unless otherwise noted, all Scripture quotations in this publication are from the *Holy Bible: New International Version* (NIV). Copyright © 1973, 1978, 1984, International Bible Society. Used by permission of Zondervan Bible Publishers. Another version used is the *King James Version* (KJV).

Printed in the United States of America

Contents

We dedicate this book
to our own families
and to the patients and families
we have had the privilege of serving
when they were making
the most difficult decisions
of their lives.

Authors

Robert D. Orr, M.D., practiced family medicine for eighteen years and was named Vermont Family Doctor of the Year in 1989. He has served on the Ethics Committee of the Vermont State Medical Society and the Ethics Commission of the Christian Medical and Dental Society. He is currently Director of Clinical Ethics and Associate Professor of Family Medicine at Loma Linda University Medical Center in California.

David L. Schiedermayer, M.D., is a Wisconsin internist and clinical ethicist. He is currently chairman of the Ethics Commission of the Christian Medical and Dental Society. He is widely published in medical and Christian ethics literature.

David B. Biebel, D.Min., is the New England Regional Director for the Christian Medical and Dental Society. He has fourteen years of pastoral experience, has authored two books, and co-authored a third.

Before You Begin

The opinions expressed are those of the authors and do not necessarily represent those of the institutions or foundations with whom they are associated. Portions of this text are adapted from Dr. Schiedermayer's columns entitled "Biblical Perspectives in Clinical Ethics," in the *Christian Medical and Dental Society Journal,* 1986-1989, and the following articles: "The Common Clinical Trilemma in Alzheimer's: Reflections on Tube Feeding and Antibiotics after a House Call to Velma D," in the *Journal of Alzheimer's Disease and Related Disorders,* and "Choices in Plague Time," in *Christianity Today.* Used with permission.

Words and phrases that appear in bold italic type can be found in the glossary on pages 199-202.

Chapter One

Medical Ethics: Everyone's Problem

"The doctor says Mother is critically ill. We need to decide if she should go on a kidney machine. What should we do?" Sandy asked her husband.

The urgency of her question pulled him from an article about fetal brain tissues being used for transplantation into the brains of patients with Parkinson's disease. "I don't know, Sandy. Will she really die if she doesn't receive dialysis?"

THE BASICS OF WISE CHOICES

More often than you might wish, medical issues touch your personal life. Perhaps someone you love is facing a serious or chronic illness. Perhaps you have a friend who's just been diagnosed with cancer. You may have recently received bad medical news yourself. Or you may be carrying the painful burden of infertility. Many of us have parents who are aged and infirm. And all of us can anticipate future deaths in our families—deaths occurring, perhaps, after a period of intensive care or prolonged hospitalization.

Every day, medical issues make the news. Perhaps today it was the latest legal battle related to frozen embryos, or something to do with abortion, or another Baby Doe situation, or another right-to-die bill, or the latest information on AIDS. Many Christians have opinions about these issues, but why they believe what they do is not clear to them, nor do most understand how these key social concerns relate to the teachings and principles of the Bible.

Where do you turn for help if you want to form a biblically sound and intellectually defensible opinion? How can you decide among perplexing alternatives? How can you prepare yourself for the eventualities all of us will face?

Sometimes Christians seem to prefer their world painted in black or white. But medical decision-making involves working in areas which are mostly gray. Many believers leave the decisions to the doctors until (and even after) they are touched by a particular issue. The problem with such a lack of involvement is that medical decisions require practical action. Not to decide in certain cases is really to decide, and such indecision may result in much unnecessary stress and guilt. Christians need to be pro-active and participate in discussions and decisions. Furthermore, when patients are involved in decisions about their own health care, they do better. They feel—and are—less helpless.

While we can't always offer resolutions to these difficult problems of living and dying, we can offer guidance where possible and suggestions where helpful, based on our personal and professional experience with medical ethics and the issues of suffering.

We have been at the bedsides of patients, parishioners, and family members, and we know these issues are deeply emotional and personal. In fact, because we consider ourselves patients as well as professionals, we are personally involved with these issues. We have not emphasized theoretical perspectives or philosophical arguments. Instead, we have focused on what is useful, practical, and rich in reality. We've tried to stay within the framework of that larger reality within which we live and move and have our being—our faith-relationship with the living God.

Instead of dispensing formulas and solutions, we invite you to enter into these issues with us, to think about and grapple with these issues for yourself. While this process requires more energy, it will strengthen your confidence and convince you that however lofty "ethics" may sound, they are basically about truth as it intersects our lives. And because of that, learning about ethics can never be very far from learning about that lofty One who is the Source of truth, who intersected life so comprehensively that purely human wisdom simply pales by comparison.

THE WISDOM OF SOLOMON

We have an opportunity to see from Scripture the wisdom of Solomon, a great man of God:

> The king said, "This one says, 'My son is alive and your son is dead,' while that one says, 'No! Your son is dead and mine is alive.'"
> Then the king said, "Bring me a sword." So they brought a sword for the king. He then gave an order: "Cut the living child in two and give half to one and half to the other."
> The woman whose son was alive was filled with compassion for her son and said to the king, "Please, my lord, give her the living baby! Don't kill him!"
> But the other said, "Neither I nor you shall have him. Cut him in two!"
> Then the king gave his ruling: "Give the living baby to the first woman. Do not kill him; she is his mother."

When all Israel heard the verdict the king had
given, they held the king in awe, because they saw that
he had wisdom from God to administer justice. (1 Kings
3:23-28)

Solomon had God's wisdom. He leaned on God in his decisions, as we see in 1 Kings 3:9: "So give your servant a discerning heart to govern your people and to distinguish between
right and wrong. For who is able to govern this great people
of yours?" God promises to give us wisdom if we ask (Psalm
32:8-10, 73:24; Proverbs 2:6-10; James 1:5-8).

Solomon's first documented "wise decision" illustrates principles important in medical decision-making. He organized his
thinking around ethical principles and a logical framework that
are still applicable today. These ethical principles are:

- Seeking to do good (beneficence)
- Avoiding harm (nonmaleficence)
- Respect for persons (autonomy)
- Giving to each his or her right or due (justice)

Solomon was faced with the decision of what to do with
a baby claimed by two mothers. He wanted to do good, while
respecting the persons involved, by giving the son to his right-
ful mother; he wanted to avoid harm by not giving the child to
the wrong mother (the sword was only a threat to help him
discern the actual mother); and he wanted to promote justice
(giving the actual mother her due).

FROM THRONE ROOM TO CLINIC

We can apply the above ethical and timeless principles in
medical decision-making today, too. And other ethical considerations also apply. (Some ethicists believe that these considerations are not principles in and of themselves but are
included in the principle of beneficence.)

Confidentiality

Confidentiality, or keeping secret the personal information learned about the patient in the context of the professional relationship, is an ancient concept. It is one of the tenets of the Oath of Hippocrates (370 BC). Sometimes the law requires some breaches of confidentiality, such as in cases of child abuse, impaired airplane pilots or bus drivers, or persons with contagious diseases or gunshot wounds. Also, some sharing of information is allowable when consultants and insurance companies are asked to pay the costs. However, if a nurse "shares" with her prayer group the intimate personal details of a patient she is caring for in the hospital so that they can pray along with her, she has broken this professional duty of confidentiality.

Telling the Truth

Each patient has the right to know the truth about his or her condition. Up until only a few years ago it was common for physicians to withhold the truth or even lie to patients if they felt that "knowing the whole truth might be harmful." Since the 1960s, truth-telling has become the norm, although it is still generally agreed among doctors that there is no moral obligation to force the truth on patients who do not want to hear it.

Sometimes people are not ready or willing to face the full truth about their case, so doctors often will tell them only what they need or want to know. For instance, Dr. Evans informed Mr. Davison that his lung cancer may be returning, even after months of chemotherapy and radiation. But the doctor never put a time frame on the case until the patient forced the issue. "How long, doctor . . . do you think we have left?" With measured words, and as sensitively as he could, Dr. Evans replied, "Sometimes certain people respond well to other treatment options, living as long as another year. But usually, I would say four to six months." Mr. Davison seemed to accept this quite calmly, but later the doctor received an angry call from Mrs. Davison who was livid about Dr. Evans "placing such negative thoughts in her husband's mind."

Christians are committed to "knowing the truth" (John 8:32) and to "speaking the truth in love" (Ephesians 4:15) in their relationships with each other. While knowing the truth is the only way to be properly oriented to reality, we temper telling the truth in love. In providing the patient with pertinent facts, proper timing, the choice of words, and the person's emotional state are all important considerations. In discussing the manner in which a patient is told the facts about diagnosis and prognosis, one ethicist has noted, "It is important to remember that not only is there a moral rule against deception, there is also one against causing pain. Thus, the way in which one tells the truth is not morally irrelevant."[1]

Truth-telling is related to respect for persons (autonomy), since if we truly respect another, we will relate to him or her honestly and forthrightly. Also, since autonomy includes the patient's making treatment decisions on the recommendation of the doctor, it is essential that the patient know as many facts as possible.

Sanctity of Life

Sanctity of life is the principle that human life has inestimable value. Paul Ramsey, a Christian ethicist, interprets this principle to mean that an individual human life is "absolutely unique, inviolable, irreplaceable, noninterchangeable, not substitutable, and not meldable with other lives."[2]

Thus, the value of a human life does not consist in its worth to anybody, but is intrinsic; there can be no degrees of value and no comparison of the value of different individual's lives regardless of their medical or social condition. An elderly patient's life is as valuable as a young patient's life. Until only recently, the sanctity of life was the primary principle of ethics in medicine. Even though this principle derived from the Bible's teaching that God made man in His own image (Genesis 1:27), it was accepted and adhered to by unbelievers as well as believers.

Many who believe strongly in the sanctity of life are apprehensive about any discussion of quality of life. Their fear is justifiable, because quality of life has been used by some to defend utilitarian decisions based on social worth (e.g., Nazi doctors used this argument as they decided which lives were "not worth living"). As we seek the patient's good (beneficence) and recognize the inherent worth of the individual (sanctity of life), we cannot ignore the patient's overall condition. Leon Kass said it well: "I think one can walk between the extremes of vitalism and 'quality control,' and uphold in so doing the respect that life itself commands for itself."[3]

Medical ethics is about the collision of principles and values with a broken and fallen world. In this conflict, the sanctity of life principle can guide Christians who affirm that, as persons made in God's image, people of all ages (from before birth to the very old) are of inestimable value and therefore worthy of the greatest honor. Because this principle is so foundational for believers, it impacts most of the clinical ethical decisions we face. For this reason, we visualize it as the foundation of our *principles in biblical clinical ethics*:

- Doing good (beneficence)
- Avoiding harm (nonmaleficence)
- Respect for persons (autonomy)
- Giving to each person his due (justice)
- Keeping secrets (confidentiality)
- Telling the truth (veracity)
- The sanctity of life (every person is worthy of honor)

In addition, several other factors affect medical decisions.

Medical Futility
Medical futility is difficult to define. Some physicians and patients would consider treatment to be futile if it does not have a good possibility of returning the patient to a desired

level of health. Others call it "futile" only when it is nearly guaranteed that the proposed treatment will effect no improvement at all.

The key question is the treatment goal: What is it? And how likely is it that this goal will be achieved? Once these questions are addressed, the pivotal issue becomes the value placed by the patient on the possible gain.[4]

In terms of a biblical perspective, life itself seems futile unless our human frailty is linked to the strength of faith in God (see Ecclesiastes). In contrast to the inner, eternal spiritual life that results from belief in God, all medical treatment is ultimately futile, since all will physically die. Even Lazarus, raised from the dead by Jesus (John 11:38-44), eventually died again. On the other hand, Jesus must have thought that for His friend to be physically alive was preferable to his remaining dead, and He must not have considered Lazarus' healing as futile.

When believers encounter the question of medical futility, we must remember that our lives are in God's hands and that whatever treatment medicine offers, it only aids the healing that must come from Him. As Ambroise Paré, a noted sixteenth-century French surgeon, wrote, "I bandaged them, but God he healeth them."[5] Faith finds its ultimate peace in trusting the sovereign plan of the Almighty God, while recognizing that "there is a time to die." Prayer helps in discerning if now is that time.

For many people dealing with death, however, medicine is a substitute for God. They strive by whatever methods and technologies science has developed to stave off the inevitable, if even for a few more days or hours. Such efforts are futile.

Costs or Allocation of Resources
We are called to be good stewards of our financial blessings, and observers of America's medical care system have noted both its generosity and its injustice. Since cost constraints are becoming increasingly important in clinical practice, we are accountable

for the way in which we spend our health care dollars.

Cost considerations can also be justice considerations when someone has to decide who will receive the benefit of technologies when only limited funds are available or when there are millions of uninsured or indigent people.

Specific data on the cost of providing many therapies are available, and we should take such information into account when we make our decisions.

THE PRINCIPLES AT WORK

Doing Good

Mrs. Williams is a seventy-year-old woman who has had Alzheimer's disease for eight years. For the last several years, she has required *tube feeding* because she has been unable to eat. Her daughter cares for her at home. Mrs. Williams frequently develops pneumonias, but she is hospitalized for intravenous antibiotics only when liquid antibiotics fail to control her fever.

Although Mrs. Williams does not speak, she is aware of pain when she is turned in bed (to prevent bedsores). She seems also to be aware of the pleasure of being bathed. She receives weekly visits from a home health care nurse, and her doctor makes a house call every two or three months.

Mrs. Williams' case, which we will discuss later in this book, exemplifies the principle of *beneficence,* or doing good. Mrs. Williams is simply unable to care for herself. She is not terminally ill and not suffering (except for brief periods). She is being cared for by her daughter, a nurse, and a doctor; they, like good Samaritans (see Luke 10:10-37), are taking care of someone who cannot take care of herself.

The good Samaritan, Jesus said, felt compassion and came to the injured man, bandaged his wounds, pouring oil and wine on them; then he brought him to an inn and took care of him. Like the good Samaritan, health professionals "bind up the wounded" compassionately.

Christian families, nurses, and physicians can be realists, for they know the fallen state of the world. But they also know that Jesus cared and died for this world, and that He regarded each person as having intrinsic value, no matter what his disease. Beneficence, as He demonstrated, is tangible and compelling evidence of God's love, so that others might come to see and believe in Him. Jesus said to His followers, "I tell you the truth, whatever you did for one of the least of these brothers of mine, you did for me" (Matthew 25:40).

Avoiding Harm

Mrs. Rockwell is eighty-seven years old and has heart failure due to heart valve disease. She is able to move around her house, but any exertion, such as stair-climbing or lifting, makes her extremely short of breath. She has swelling of both legs for which her physician has been giving her medications, but the treatment is not very effective anymore. An *echocardiogram* (ultrasound) of the heart shows that the valves need replacement if Mrs. Rockwell is to be restored to better health.

Mrs. Rockwell's physician looked at the ultrasound report on her desk. Should she refer Mrs. Rockwell to a heart surgeon? She telephoned a heart surgeon and discussed the case with him. She learned that Mrs. Rockwell would have a thirty-five percent chance of dying during or just after surgery. Surgery could, however, restore Mrs. Rockwell to a much higher activity level.

Nonmaleficence means not harming the patient unduly. Of course, some small amount of pain is sometimes necessary in even routine medical care. Drawing blood hurts a little, but the information learned far outweighs the harm of penetrating the skin with a needle. In Mrs. Rockwell's case, however, surgery holds potential for doing great harm. She may die from the surgery. Yet if she does not have the surgery, she will avoid the immediate high risk of dying but will continue to be restricted in her activity.

Nonmaleficence is a crucial principle in medical ethics and practice. Every physician and every patient should weigh the "risks versus the benefits" of proposed treatments to determine if they might do more harm than good.

Jesus pointed out that people must consider the costs of their actions:

"Or suppose a king is about to go to war against another king. Will he not first sit down and consider whether he is able with ten thousand men to oppose the one coming against him with twenty thousand? If he is not able, he will send a delegation while the other is still a long way off and will ask for terms of peace." (Luke 14:31-33)

If a procedure can only do harm, it must, of course, be avoided. If there is some potential for good, even with great risk of harm, the patient should be the key figure in making the value-laden decision of whether the proposed treatment is worthwhile.

Medical futility is also involved in Mrs. Rockwell's case. At what point does heart surgery become futile? Some think that this procedure would be futile if Mrs. Rockwell's chances of dying become greater than a given number, perhaps ninety percent. Others would argue that if Mrs. Rockwell wants the surgery, despite the risk, it cannot be futile since it has value to her.

Respect for Persons

Mr. Meyer, a sixty-two-year-old recently retired man, sees his physician, complaining of stomach pain and weight loss. An x-ray shows that cancer of the colon is the cause of his pain and weight loss. His wife and physician agree not to tell him, and he is scheduled for surgery. At the time of surgery, he is found to have widely spread cancer. Mr. Meyer is not told of the findings and consequently he does not participate in any of the decisions about his future care.

Sick people have the same interest as healthy people in

being involved in decisions about their lives. The principle of *autonomy,* or self-determination, is a matter of honoring the patient. As patients, our free will should be respected; doctors and nurses should not keep secrets from us. They should *tell us the truth.*

God informs us and lets us decide about various issues as a matter of principle. For example, His will is for all to be saved through faith in Jesus Christ (2 Peter 3:9), but He doesn't force us to be saved. If we know the choices before us, understand the gospel, and reject it, we will perish. This same principle is in operation on a day-to-day level as well. God informs us of our choices through His Word. We can choose to trust and obey or not.

If God grants us free will regarding the issue of our souls, using words to communicate the choices, then how much more should physicians give their patients free will over their bodies, using words to communicate their choices. It is true that we are not our own—we are bought with a price (1 Corinthians 6:19-20). But the biblical perspective of free will allows us to make our own medical decisions. Patients deserve honor as persons. Jesus put it this way in Matthew 22:39-40: "Love your neighbor as yourself. All the Law and the Prophets hang on these two commandments" (loving God and neighbor).

Justice
Mr. Roper, twenty-five years old, is admitted to the hospital with severe liver failure. After running some tests, his doctor determines that he is dying and that the only way to save him is to perform a liver transplantation. However, Mr. Roper has no money. The transplant surgeon is willing to perform the operation for free, but the hospital administrators say they can't afford to pay for the hospital costs of the transplant.

Economic issues are increasingly important in the ethics of health care. *Justice,* or giving to each person their due, is an important principle in any health care system. Does justice in Mr. Roper's case mean giving him a new liver? Is this his due?

Justice is a crucial biblical and ethical principle. We read in Micah 6:8, "He has showed you, O man, what is good. And what does the LORD require of you? To act justly and to love mercy and to walk humbly with your God." Justice is required in human relationships and in medical ethics. In the case of Mr. Roper, the justice issues are complex, because while Mr. Roper should be allowed the chance to live, justice must weigh whether public support of his transplant operation should take precedence over public support of other goods, such as immunizations, prenatal care, etc.; in other words, there is an allocation of resources question.

Within the current medical system, hospitals don't make such trade-offs directly (spending money on one patient never directly shortchanges another in a nonsocialist, nonclosed system). Nonetheless, spending money on Mr. Roper's transplant would indirectly take money away from other programs. If organs are in short supply, the justice issue becomes even more difficult. Who gets the liver when Mr. Roper and another patient both need it? To whom is it due—Mr. Roper, a twenty-five-year-old single and unemployed man, or Mr. Olson, a fifty-year-old father of four, a successful businessman, and a church deacon? If our answer comes quickly, "Mr. Olson," how do we decide that we have "done justice"?

DIFFERENT WAYS OF MAKING ETHICAL DECISIONS

There are a number of frameworks for acting upon principles in medical decisions. Contemporary medical ethics include four broad schools of thought, each jousting with the others for dominance.[6]

Ethical Frameworks
- Duties/principles (Deontological)
- Consequences (Utilitarianism)
- Process (Moral Analysis)
- Language (Moral Discourse)

Duties/Principles

The first school, and the one with which many Christians are comfortable, is reflected in the works of Paul Ramsey and in his book *The Patient as Person*.[7] Ramsey emphasizes the importance of firm moral rules (or duties), and he urges adherence to traditional medical and moral principles. Rejecting "situation ethics" (which we shall discuss in a moment), he insists that some features of moral acts other than their outcome determine whether they are right or wrong.

Because of its emphasis on sense of duty, this approach is called the *deontological* theory of ethics (from the Greek word deon, meaning *duty*). Lying, for example, is wrong even if it may result in positive consequences.

Suppose that in the case of Mr. Meyer, the patient's wife feared that telling him the diagnosis of cancer would make him despair, lose hope, and die. Lying to Mr. Meyer about his diagnosis might then result in a longer life. The deontologic system of ethics would argue that such a lie is wrong even if it might do the patient some good; it is wrong because, in general, lying is wrong.

Consequences

The second school is represented by philosopher Joseph Fletcher, author of *Morals and Medicine*.[8] Fletcher is the father of what has been called "situation ethics," a system which rejects fixed moral rules and principles in favor of context and consequences. Situation ethics looks at the specific needs and life circumstances of the patients and considers each case individually. The advantage of this system is its flexibility.

Situation ethics is an example of *utilitarianism,* which seeks to define morally appropriate actions by the nonmoral value (knowledge, pleasure, wealth) they produce. These theories are sometimes called *teleological* (from the Greek word *telos,* meaning *ends*), because it says the outcome of an action determines its moral usefulness. Lying to Mr. Meyer would then be justified if it could be proven that he would actually benefit from the lie, perhaps either by living longer or by having a better life during his remaining time.

Process

A third school, composed of moral philosophers like Daniel Callahan and Arthur Caplan, draws on the language of secular philosophy, clarifying and analyzing moral problems, concerned more with process than with the outcome of actual individual cases. This approach is called moral analysis.

Analysis of Mr. Meyer's case would result in arguments to clarify the nature of the lie and the rationale for lying. This approach may be very helpful in specific kinds of cases where the issues are difficult to pinpoint and where the outcomes are unknown or unknowable. In Mr. Meyer's case, most moral philosophers would urge that he be told the truth even if it might result in some potential harm.

Language

A fourth group of ethicists, discouraged with the current state of *moral discourse,* have tried to find a new language with which to speak about medical-ethical issues. Alastair MacIntyre writes about virtue, William F. May about covenant, James M. Gustafson about fidelity, Robert Veatch and Tristin Engelhardt about partnership and personal autonomy.

These ethicists would redefine what is at stake in Mr. Meyer's case and evaluate whether telling the truth would be virtuous, whether it would keep an unwritten covenant with the patient and show fidelity and partnership, and whether patient autonomy requires truth-telling.

SOLOMON'S FRAMEWORK OF ETHICS

When Solomon employed the principles of beneficence, nonmaleficence, autonomy, and justice in deciding to pretend to divide the baby and create a situation in which he could discern the women's motives, his framework was *deontological* (he would not have killed the baby in any case). He would have obeyed the principle in Deuteronomy 5:17, "You shall not murder." But he wisely gathered information as well.

He was considered a wise decision-maker by the people, because his process was good (he sought God for wisdom and redefined the situation so he could discern the truth), and the outcome was also just (the right woman received her due, as did the child).

Organizing our thinking, gathering information, and asking God for wisdom can provide us with ethical solutions to the sometimes complex problems we and our family members face.

FOR DISCUSSION

The best way to see how ethical principles really work is to meet with a few other people and discuss what you would do in a specific case. We have provided a variety of cases, and we suggest that instead of trying to cover them all, you will benefit most by choosing the one or two that seem most relevant or challenging and then spending your time examining these from many angles.

Opening: The natural human tendency in discussions is to say the polite or safe thing. But in order to have truly fruitful interaction about issues in medical ethics, we encourage you to trust each other and God enough to risk saying what you really think.

It will help if you know something about each other's backgrounds in terms of medical decision-making. For instance, one group member may have cared for an ill relative at home. Another may have experienced a long hospitalization. A third may be infertile. Each of these persons will have some special insights to contribute.

So before launching into discussion of these cases, give each group member an opportunity to briefly describe one medical ethical decision that he or she has had to face in the past few years. It could be something as simple as whether or not to have a certain test, or as heart-wrenching as working through the slow death of a loved one.

1. Eight-year-old Josh has a *congenital* kidney and bone disease. Three kidney transplants have failed, and he has had multiple severe complications. He is now on *dialysis*. He screams in pain each time blood is drawn or the dialysis needle is inserted. He sometimes asks the doctor to stop dialysis. His parents are torn between the desire to keep him alive and the wish to see his suffering end. Josh's father confides, in addition, that Josh's care is nearly bankrupting the family.
    a. How does the principle of sanctity of life apply here? Does this principle mean we can never stop treatment?
    b. What role should cost have in this case? Is further dialysis of Josh medically futile?
    c. How would you treat Josh? Would you stop dialysis? Could death (which would occur fairly soon and without much pain) ever be seen as in his best interest? Explain your reasoning.
    d. Read the story of David's response to his own critically ill child (2 Samuel 12:12-23). How might this apply to Josh's case? (Note: We'll examine the problems of chronic care and "pulling the plug" again in chapters 8 and 9.)

2. Mr. Meyer, the man whose doctor and wife agreed not to tell him of his colon cancer, becomes progressively more ill. All of his visitors, including his eight-year-old grandson, are cautioned not to tell him his diagnosis.
    a. The principles of autonomy and of truth-telling are violated here because of the wishes of Mr. Meyer's wife. Why do you think she wanted to keep his diagnosis a secret?
    b. Lying is wrong, and it also usually has harmful effects on patients. What harm could come to Mr. Meyer because

of this lie? Why should doctors have to ask patients for consent to procedures? (Note: We'll look more closely at "informed consent" in chapter 5.)

3. In medical school, a common principle taught is, "First of all, do no harm." Some Christians might object, saying the primary rule should be, "First of all, the image of God." This is another way of saying, "First of all, the sanctity of life."
   a. Which rule do you think should be primary, and why?
   b. How might many of the issues in medical ethics be framed differently if the latter perspective regained preeminence?
   c. Do you think it is possible, in today's world, for the latter perspective to become primary? Why, or why not?

4. If you agree that the sanctity of life is a fundamental principle in medical ethics, what can you do to promote this aspect of the Kingdom's viewpoint? You may want to come back to this question periodically as you work through upcoming chapters.

NOTES:
1. Bernard Gert and Charles M. Culver, "Moral Theory in Neurologic Practice," *Seminars in Neurology*, March 1984, 4(1):9-14.
2. Paul Ramsey, quoted in "On Paul Ramsey" by David H. Smith, *Second Opinion*, vol. 6, November 1987.
3. Leon Kass, *Toward a More Natural Science* (New York: The Free Press, 1985).
4. John D. Lantos, et al., "The Illusion of Futility in Clinical Practice," *The American Journal of Medicine*, July 1989, 87:81-84.
5. Erwin H. Ackerknecht, M.D., *A Short History of Medicine* (Baltimore, MD: Johns Hopkins University Press, 1982), p. 111.
6. Daniel Callahan, "Shattuck Lecture: Comtemporary Biomedical Ethics," *New England Journal Medicine*, May 29, 1980, 302(22):1228-1233.
7. Paul Ramsey, *The Patient as Person: Explorations in Medical Ethics* (New Haven: Yale University Press, 1970).
8. Joseph F. Fletcher, *Morals and Medicine* (Boston: Beacon Press, 1954), deals with the moral problems of the patient's right to know the truth, contraception, artificial insemination, sterilization, and euthanasia.

Chapter Two

Making Sarah Laugh

"Abe?" Sarah asked softly, not wanting to wake her husband if he was already asleep.

"What, dear?" Abe muttered as he came out of dreamland.

"Oh, I was just wondering," Sarah continued. "Just lying here and wondering what we should do with the extra ones."

"Extra ones? What extra ones?" Abe replied.

"Well . . . the extra fertilized eggs—what did the doctor call them? *Embryos*, that's it. What do you think they usually do with the extra embryos they don't use?"

"I don't know," Abe said with a yawn. "But you could find out easily enough in the morning. Just call the doctor."

Early the next morning, the answer Sarah received forced her to stop and think.

"Well," Dr. Michaels paused, quickly considering his patient's background and their history together. "In this clinic, usually the leftover *zygotes* are discarded, unless other arrangements are made. Of course," he quickly added, "we need to remember that even in natural reproduction as many as fifty to seventy-five percent are also lost."

Now, as she sat at the breakfast bar, Sarah reviewed the whole process she and Abe had been through in these past three years. It was a process of trying to achieve what all their friends were accomplishing without a second thought: having a baby, their own baby.

Just thinking through all the procedures and techniques they had tried so far—not to mention fifteen thousand dollars they had spent—brought back the pain again, the aching pain of longing to be a mother. The additional thought of those "leftover" embryos being flushed down the drain by some disinterested lab technician did nothing to relieve her distress. Her nagging sense of emptiness and incompetence almost bordered on despair.

Dr. Michaels, it had seemed, was the first person to really understand and accept the anguish Abe and Sarah shared. Since their marriage ten years earlier, they had been trying to achieve something that was supposed to happen naturally. Only gradually had they concluded that the problem was not due to poor timing, stress, or bad luck. It was due to infertility.

TRYING TO HAVE A BABY

Artificial Insemination-Homologous (AIH)

For the first year, Dr. Michaels had prescribed various hormones, none of which brought about conception. Then, after Sarah's x-rays showed no *fallopian tube* disease, he had suggested the next step, artificial insemination, using sperm that Abe would provide. The technique was called *artificial insemination-homologous* (AIH). The doctor informed Sarah and Abe that the technology for AIH had been used for more than thirty years.

Since AIH requires masturbation or the use of a condom

during intercourse for the collection of sperm, Dr. Michaels had inquired, for the first and only time, whether their religious convictions would prohibit pursuing this new course of action. As far as Abe and Sarah knew, neither their church nor their denomination had published anything about it.

Once they had decided to go ahead with AIH, the technology available posed another question: "Would they like to select a boy or girl?" There are methods of *X and Y sperm isolation* that could give them this choice, Dr. Michaels explained. Although Abe was eager to have a son, they decided against this option. Somehow it seemed to take the whole thing out of the hands of God.

Gamete Intra-Fallopian Transfer (GIFT)
After several failed attempts using AIH, Dr. Michaels suggested another method, called GIFT (*gamete* intra-fallopian transfer), which promised a success rate as high as thirty percent. A relatively new procedure that transfers both sperm and egg into the woman's fallopian tube, this technique also required either masturbation or the use of a condom to collect sperm after intercourse. In addition, it required that Sarah undergo *laparoscopy*. Again, the couple ruled out gender selection, and again, to their growing disappointment, this procedure was unsuccessful.

So now, even though they had rejected the idea earlier, they began to consider another option: artificial insemination using sperm from a donor.

Artificial Insemination by Donor (AID)
Dr. Michaels explained that AID had been used successfully in the conception and birth of more than 250,000 children in the United States alone. Of course, this method would introduce a third party into the process of having a child. Sarah had expressed strong reservations about the selection of a donor and the need to keep the child's origin a secret.

But, they reasoned, AID would allow them to have a child

with a genetic link to at least one of them. So, with Abe's consent, they went ahead, using cryopreserved (frozen) sperm from a donor (who, by the way, had tested negative for the deadly AIDS virus six months after donation).

This procedure, too, had been unsuccessful. It led them to the most recent attempt, which involved a technique resulting in Sarah's embryo dilemma: *in-vitro fertilization* (IVF).

In-Vitro Fertilization (IVF)

Dr. Michaels had explained that IVF is effective in overcoming many infertility problems. This technique allows the direct contact of sperm and egg in a test tube, and permits a wider range of possibilities. These include the use of donor sperm or donor eggs if the couple involved is unable to provide them. This would introduce not only a third party, but potentially a fourth, into the process of having a child.

The doctor mentioned that if Abe produced markedly abnormal sperm, or if there were some history of genetic disease, donor sperm might be used. Or sperm from a donor might be used as a backup if fertilization had not occurred within twelve to eighteen hours after the exposure of Sarah's eggs to Abe's sperm. Additionally, if he should find it impossible to retrieve eggs from Sarah, Dr. Michaels said they might have the option of using eggs from a donor—possibly another woman undergoing IVF whose menstrual cycle coincided with Sarah's and who had excess eggs.

The fertilization of Sarah's eggs by Abe's sperm had been successful, but implantation in Sarah had been unsuccessful.

Following confirmation of yet another failure of modern medicine to help Abe and Sarah become parents, Dr. Michaels had suggested they consider the final technologies available to help them have their own child: surrogate embryo transfer (SET) and surrogate motherhood. He also mentioned that they would need to decide what to do with the unused frozen embryos, a decision that could wait until they recovered from their most recent disappointment.

Finally, the doctor also suggested they begin the process of adoption.

Assessing the Situation

Now, as Sarah sat reviewing the entire experience, she felt bombarded with numerous conflicting thoughts and emotions. In the process of trying to have a child, she, Abe, and Dr. Michaels had created numerous embryos that all failed to survive, even when implanted in her own body. The extra frozen embryos might now be unceremoniously discarded unless an alternate plan were to be made. The newspaper had recently reported a custody case involving seven frozen embryos of a now-divorced couple. Custody was awarded to the mother, whose intention was to use the embryos to become pregnant. If successful, the father might be required to pay child support. Sarah wondered whether the embryos she and Abe had formed together were really like children.

Was it her fault that she was infertile? Abe's fault? Wasn't some of this God's responsibility?

Certainly their motivations had been commendable. Could there be any higher goal than to desire a child of their own to love and nurture, whom they would try to raise to become a responsible member of society?

Suddenly, Sarah reached for the phone. She wouldn't give up the dream. After all, they had tried the other techniques which had failed, so why not continue until there were no more options? Dialing her best friend Heather, she explained to Heather the procedure of surrogate embryo transfer (SET). She implored her help in what seemed to be an impossible situation. Heather agreed.

Surrogate Embryo Transfer (SET)

After refraining from coitus for several days before *ovulation*, Heather was artificially inseminated with Abe's sperm. They understood that if this procedure was unsuccessful, the option remained to try again, using donor sperm.

Five days after the insemination (after five days of surrogate *gestational* motherhood), the embryo was washed out of
Heather's uterus and transferred to Sarah's uterus. Heather
knew from the beginning that if the embryo could not be
washed out of her uterus, she would either have to carry the
child to term or have an abortion.

Sarah's uterus was ready for the embryo, because the ovu-
lations of the two women had been synchronized by the use of
hormones. The option also existed to freeze the embryo for a
time in case Sarah was not ready.

The SET procedure was also unsuccessful on several occasions. Each time Sarah had a miscarriage, and finally, unable
to face further heartache with this method, Sarah and Abe
again turned to Heather for help in having a child.

Surrogate Motherhood (SM)
Still willing to help, Heather signed a contract giving Abe and
Sarah custody of the child if the procedure was successful.
This procedure seemed simply an extension of SET, which
they had already tried several times. Abe's sperm were again
used to artificially inseminate Heather. She became pregnant
and delivered a healthy baby boy.

In the meantime, two things happened. Abe and Sarah
were approved as adoptive parents, and Sarah discovered she
was pregnant. .

Adoption (A)
Adoption, granting full familial privileges to a genetically unre-
lated child, has been the time-honored method for an infertile
couple to have a child. The new reproductive technologies have
made adoption less desirable to many couples, because they
offer an opportunity to produce a genetically related child
and/or experience the birth process. Moreover, legalization
and social acceptance of abortion have made adoption more
difficult for the infertile couple, because far fewer babies are
available than in previous generations.

INFERTILITY AND MODERN MEDICINE

Infertility is an age-old problem. Perhaps you recognized our fictionalized story as a modernized version of the biblical story of Abraham, Sarah, and Hagar (Genesis 16:1–21:3).

Infertility is common. Twenty percent of all couples seek professional consultation to increase their chances of having a baby.[1] Those who have not experienced infertility may fail to realize the trauma experienced by modern Sarahs and Abrahams. According to one study, the stress of infertility is second only to the stress caused by the death of a loved one.[2]

Medical science attempts to relieve this suffering, using a variety of treatments. Besides hormonal and surgical therapies, which have proven helpful to many couples, there are many new reproductive technologies available.

In fact, there are now twenty-four ways to have children, depending on the source of sperm or egg, the site of fertilization, and the site of pregnancy.[3] A child can have as many as five parents; sperm from father A and an egg from mother B can be united and the embryo implanted in mother C; the child born to C could be raised by father D and mother E. Presumably one of the major problems such a child would have is deciding how many Mother's Day cards to send!

With apologies for being sarcastic, our point is that non-sexual methods of reproduction lead to an increasing complexity within childbirth—not only technologically but also in terms of lineage, legitimacy, and identity. Also, such efforts to have a genetically related child are very costly.

Many of these technologies are available only to the upper class. Some affluent infertile couples claim an absolute right to have related children since they are paying the cost. Although others challenge this absolute right from a social justice standpoint, it would be practically difficult to force reallocation of these discretionary personal monies to, say, children in the third world. Presumably, the cost is worthwhile to these couples if it alleviates their suffering.

However, there is another cost, unacceptable for some who believe that human life is sacred from the moment of conception. In the course of trying to have a baby genetically related to at least one of them, Sarah and Abe allowed the creation (and destruction) of multiple human embryos. Now the fate of several more embryos in storage also rests with them.

Finally, to assess the morality of their actions, Abe and Sarah might have gained wisdom by considering major religious traditions. As far as they knew, their Protestant church had no official stance on these issues, but Abe and Sarah never actually inquired of their pastor. And what if they had been Jewish or Catholic? Would there have been any guidelines?

RELIGIOUS TRADITIONS AND MEDICAL PROCREATION

As with so many issues, there is no monolithic unity in the Protestant church. Protestant teachings have usually been more permissive regarding birth control for married couples, masturbation, and new reproductive technologies than other religious traditions.

The Jewish Position
Religious Jews have no authoritative rabbi like the Catholic Pope to present an "official" view on new reproductive technologies. Instead, different rabbis of orthodox, conservative, and reformed synagogues interpret Jewish law differently. AID and other techniques are performed in Israel.

When formulating their position on the new technologies, rabbis have in general been concerned about three fundamental Jewish decrees:

- *Consanguinity* is sinful.
- The wasting of seed (masturbation) is sinful.
- It is a sin for a married woman to conceive by the sperm of a man not her husband.

Most Jewish scholars, however, believe that the artificial injection of the seed of a stranger is not itself an adulterous act, and thus the woman's husband is not obliged to divorce her, nor is the child illegitimate. Since the child born after AID is to be the child of the woman rather than the donor, the child belongs to the family and is Jewish. This modern position has a powerful parallel in the New Testament account of the conception and birth of Jesus, including the response of Joseph to Mary's pregnancy (Matthew 1:18-25).

The Catholic Position

The encyclicals of the Pope have always forbidden masturbation and contraception; the first decree on this topic was made in 1897. Recently, the most comprehensive Catholic reaction to reproductive technologies, *Instruction on Respect for Human Life in Its Origin and on the Dignity of Procreation,* also banned all use of reproductive technologies.[4] (See appendix B.)

The Catholic church approves of adoption, and also (possibly) of GIFT if the couple uses a perforated condom so that some sperm may escape during intercourse and make the pregnancy theoretically "natural." The remaining sperm can, according to several theologians, be placed in the fallopian tube without violation of the principles of the *Instruction.* Other church leaders, however, believe that GIFT is also forbidden by the principles of the *Instruction.* GIFT would be against the principles of the document if the condom used to collect the sperm were not perforated or if the sperm were collected by masturbation.

The Catholic position is that technology should not separate the "procreative act" from the "unitive" (sex) act. As Cardinal Bernadin of Chicago noted,

> Human beings are not God, even though we find it difficult to admit at times . . . Not all the human mind is capable of doing is worth doing. . . . we must ensure that in pursuit of treatment, the good of life is not lost . . . the fundamental meaning of life should not be violated.[5]

THE PROBLEM OF THE SLIPPERY SLOPE

The slope of human sexuality is a dangerous one; at stake is our perception of what it means to be human. Once Sarah and Abe began employing technology in an effort to reproduce, it became increasingly easy to pursue the next available method until finally the lives of Sarah, Abe, and Heather became inextricably intertwined forever.

The initial appeal of the Catholic position is that it solves the problems posed by modern reproductive technologies by basically forbidding them all. This position, however, also forecloses all possibility of doing good with knowledge that God has allowed us to possess.

The technology surrounding human reproduction is not automatically immoral. For instance, while tests of sperm count require masturbation, they may provide very useful information which can help couples have children the "natural" way.

How might Saint Thomas Aquinas have weighed the means and the ends regarding this issue? Would the masturbation be justified in order to create a life within the context of marriage?

And what about Augustine? He believed that if artificial methods of reproduction ever became available, we would be morally obligated to use them to avoid the fleshly pleasures of intercourse!

BEYOND THE SLIPPERY SLOPE

Let's go back to our real-life situation described in Scripture:

> Now Sarai, Abram's wife, had borne him no children. But she had an Egyptian maidservant named Hagar; so she said to Abram, "The LORD has kept me from having children. Go, sleep with my maidservant; perhaps I can build a family through her."
> He slept with Hagar, and she conceived.

When she knew she was pregnant, she [Hagar] began to despise her mistress. Then Sarai said to Abram, "You are responsible for the wrong I am suffering. I put my servant in your arms, and now that she knows she is pregnant, she despises me. May the LORD judge between you and me."

"Your servant is in your hands," Abram said. "Do with her whatever you think best." Then Sarai mistreated Hagar; so she fled from her. (Genesis 16:1-2,4-6)

Some reproductive "technologies" were never a good idea— specifically, surrogate motherhood. Compare our modern story:

Heather delivered a healthy son and gave him to Sarah and Abe as promised. Since giving him up, Heather has been depressed. When she learned that Sarah was pregnant, Heather retained the services of a lawyer in an attempt to regain custody of her son. A court battle ensued. Sarah and Abe argued that the contract they had Heather sign before conception entitles them to the child, which is, after all, genetically related to Abe. Heather argued that a child should never be taken from its birth mother on the basis of a contract.

Should Sarah and Abe have enlisted the help of a third party to assist them in their quest for a genetically-related child? Should the potential for lineage dispute influence our perception of the merits of various reproductive technologies? How do surrogate motherhood or surrogate embryo transfer compare to IVF or AID in terms of ethical analysis?[6] (See table 1.)

COUNSELING SARAH AND ABE

Suppose Sarah and Abe had sought our advice before starting to fall all the way down the slippery slope? Could we have helped them sort through the complex ethical, moral, and spiritual issues these technologies produce, instead of simply telling them not to try any of these techniques?

The very first thing we could have expressed is compassion for their distress. We know that infertility has been a major source of anguish through the ages—anguish clearly reflected in the pages of the Bible. (See appendix A.)

Then, after explaining the various alternatives, we could have advised them *against* surrogate motherhood and surrogate embryo transfer. Predictable and serious trouble lurks in those techniques for all parties; we have biblical precedent as well as recent experience to help us on this issue.

In terms of IVF, while we have serious problems with the lack of embryo protection as this technique is currently employed, our concerns would have lessened if Dr. Michaels were to have used safeguards for embryos and promised not to practice *eugenics* and embryo experimentation.

In relation to AID, we would have weighed the good of having a child against the ethical problems of this particular technology. This technique has worked well for many hundreds of thousands of couples, but there are potential psychological dangers to both parents and child. Also, with AID there is the potential risk of contracting one of the AIDS viruses, since screening tests for HIV infection are not one-hundred percent sensitive or specific.

We would have encouraged Abe and Sarah to pursue AIH, GIFT, and adoption, and would have pointed out the positive biblical attitude toward adoption, especially for those who are adopted with love (Romans 8:15-17).

We could have advised them to pray, knowing also that God sometimes relieves infertility as an answer to prayer. We would have listened to their concerns. And we could have put them in contact with a physician who agrees with the perspective that insofar as God has given doctors any power to assist Him in the creation of human life, this power should be prayerfully used in awe and in deference to Him.

For like God, our goal is to hear the laughter of Sarah and not the weeping of Hagar, to foster life instead of death through medical technology. But we must be cautious. Even in this endeavor we shall reap what we sow; God is not mocked.

FOR DISCUSSION

Opening: Ask for volunteers to share any personal experiences they have had with the issues of reproductive technology. For instance, have you known someone who struggled with infertility? Have you ever been asked for advice about any of these questions?

1. Suppose you are Abe and Sarah's pastor, and they come to you for advice about which technologies are acceptable. What advice will you give? What scriptural principles do you think apply?

2. Sarah is a part of your prayer group, and she has been bringing up the matter of her infertility weekly for over a year now. As one of her best friends, you:

   ___ wish she would stop bringing it up, since it makes everybody uncomfortable.
   ___ think she does it because everybody else just wants to talk about their kids all the time.
   ___ hurt with her and wish you could help.
   ___ give her the name of a Christian doctor who specializes in infertility problems.
   ___ pray that she will conceive.
   ___ other (name it).

3. In your view, is artificial insemination by donor (AID) equivalent to adultery? In preparing your answer, you may wish to review the current Jewish perspective on this topic (pages 36-37). Also, for relevant biblical cases, consider:
   a. The story of Ruth. She was the Gentile daughter-in-law of Naomi, whose kinsman Boaz redeemed Naomi's childlessness. (Naomi's sons, one of whom had been Ruth's

husband, had both died.) Boaz married Ruth, and their first child was reckoned as the heir of her deceased husband. That son, Obed, was the grandfather of King David and one of the ancestors of Jesus.

b. For a negative example of the kinsman-redeemer see Genesis 38:6-10, where Onan refuses to father offspring by his deceased brother's wife because the children would not be regarded as his own. The sin of Onan is not "spilling his seed" on the ground, but his unwillingness to fulfill his duty to his brother. This resulted in Onan, too, losing his life as judgment from God.

c. While some people view the case of Mary, Joseph, and Jesus as a parallel to surrogate motherhood, it may be closer to AID, connecting quite positively to the current Jewish practice with AID.

4. Does knowing that many, if not most, fertilized eggs fail to implant successfully in the uterus under natural conditions affect your view of reproductive technologies at all? Why, or why not?

Do you think that in Heaven there will be billions of "persons" who were never physically born because of one reason or another? Where and how do you draw the line in your own thinking regarding when these embryos achieve the status of personhood?

5. Here is a real case. In Tennessee, a formerly married couple battled over the status and ownership of frozen embryos. The husband wished to block his wife's possible use or donation of the embryos.

What would you do if you had to decide this case? Would you:

___ allow the destruction of the embryos, according to the husband's wishes?

___ allow the wife to have the embryos implanted, with

the intention of bringing one or more of them to term?

___ allow the adoption of these embryos by another couple wishing to have a child?

APPENDIX A: A BIBLICAL PERSPECTIVE ON INFERTILITY

The Bible presents infertility as a condition in which God can intervene as a result of prayer (Genesis 20:17-18, 25:21; 1 Samuel 1:11). Besides Sarah, God enabled Rebecca, Hannah, Manoah's wife, and Elizabeth to overcome the problem of infertility. Their children, Isaac, Jacob and Esau, Samuel, Samson, and John the Baptist were of critical importance in God's plan. We are told by Jesus that one of them, John the Baptist, is the greatest among men born of women (Matthew 11:11). The initial points we glean from a biblical study of infertility are:

1. Infertile couples suffer severely.
2. The inability to have children is a special scourge in some cultures (those who have lived in third world countries have seen the agony of those who are childless).
3. Some couples will try any available method to have genetically related children.
4. God sometimes relieves infertility as a result of prayer.
5. Just as God adopts us (Romans 8:15-17, 8:23; 1 Peter 1:3-5), human beings can adopt the children of others (Exodus 2:5-10, Esther 2:7).
6. The children of those previously experiencing infertility, born either through a miraculous intervention within the marriage or as a result of other arrangements, may play crucial roles in God's plan. God also uses adopted children (for example, Moses and Esther) to accomplish unique purposes.

TABLE 1 (Adapted from reference 6)

AN ETHICAL SCORING OF REPRODUCTIVE TECHNOLOGIES*

Ethical Issues	AIH	GIFT	AID	IVF	SET	SM	A
Risk	0	1	1	1	2	3	0
Embryo destruction	0	0	0	3	3	0	0
Embryo research/sale	0	0	0	3	3	0	0
Masturbation	1	1	1	1	1	1	0
Required abortion	0	0	0	0	0	4	0
Eugenic potential	1	1	2	3	3	3	0
Third party involved	0	0	2	2	3	4	1
Second family involved	0	0	1	1	3	4	1
Lineage disputes	0	0	1	1	3	4	1
Totals	2	3	8	15	21	23	3

*Scores are as follows:
1–of ethical concern;
2–of sufficient concern to require careful scrutiny;
3–of sufficient concern to discourage practice;
4–ethically problematic; procedure should be prohibited on this ground
alone

Abbreviations
AIH, GIFT, AID, IVF, SET, A, and SM (surrogate motherhood)
are defined on pages 30-34.

Description of "Ethical Issues" Terms
Risk—physical risk to any involved, from childbirth, surgery,
or infection.
Embryo destruction—potential for production of embryos that
are destroyed at a rate higher than baseline miscarriage rate
(fifty to seventy-five percent).
Embryo research/sale—potential for non-therapeutic research
or commercial exploitation of embryos.
Masturbation—manual stimulation of the male to induce ejacu-
lation is morally problematic to some.
Required abortion—likelihood of contract that mandates abortion of genetically or otherwise defective child.

Eugenic potential—potential for sex selection or for attempts to create a "super race."
Third party involved—level of involvement of third person.
Second family involved—level of involvement of another family.
Lineage disputes—potential for creating disputes over lineage and custody.

APPENDIX B:
THE OFFICIAL POSITION OF THE ROMAN CATHOLIC CHURCH

Most people agree that this represents the most conservative position on reproductive technology. As you think about each point, try to determine why you agree or disagree with it.

*Instruction on Respect for Human Life
in Its Origin and on the Dignity of Procreation*
Summary of Main Points
March 10, 1987

1. God created man in His own image and likeness.
2. Science and technology serve the human person.
3. One cannot use means and methods for transmitting human life which are allowable for plants and animals.
4. The human being is to be respected and treated as a person from the moment of conception.
5. Non-therapeutic experimentation on embryos is illicit.
6. The corpses of embryos and fetuses, whether they have been deliberately aborted or not, are to be respected.
7. It is immoral to produce human embryos which are destined to be disposed of as biological material.
8. Development of IVF has required innumerable destructions of human embryos.
9. The abortion mentality, which made IVF and embryo

transfer, could result in a system of radical eugenics (the attempt to make a "better man").

10. The conjugal act, willed by God, must include both the unitive and the procreative meaning.

11. Contraception deprives the conjugal act of procreative meaning.

12. Masturbation deprives procreation of the dignity which is proper to it.

13. Even AIH is therefore immoral.

14. All other new reproductive technologies are also immoral; surrogate motherhood sets up, to the detriment of families, a division between physical, psychological, and moral elements of families.

15. The suffering caused by infertility in marriage is an opportunity for sharing in a particular way in the Lord's cross, and a potential source of spiritual fruitfulness. Infertile spouses may share in adoption and assistance to other families and poor or handicapped children.

NOTES:
1. M. C. Horn and W. D. Mosher, "Use of Services for Family Planning and Infertility: United States, 1982," *Advance Data from Vital and Health Statistics*, no. 103 (Hyattsville, MD: Public Health Services, 1984), pp. 1-8.
2. Ellen W. Freeman, Andrea S. Bozer, and Karl Rickels, et al., "Psychological Evaluation and Support in a Program of In-Vitro Fertilization and Embryo Transfer," *Fertility and Sterility*, January 1985, 43:48-52.
3. David D. Weaver and Luis F. Escobar, "Twenty-Four Ways to Have Children," *American Journal of Medical Genetics*, March 1987, 26:737-740.
4. "Instruction on Respect for Human Life in Its Origin and on the Dignity of Procreation," *Origins*, NC Documentary Service 16, March 19, 1987, pp. 698-711.
5. Joseph Cardinal Bernadin, AOA Lecture, Pritzker School of Medicine, University of Chicago, April 29, 1987.
6. Sherman Elias and George J. Annas, "Social Policy Considerations in Non-coital Reproduction," *Journal of the American Medical Association*, January 3, 1986, 255(1):62-68.

Mommy's Rights, Baby's Rights

"Place it in a basin, cover it with a towel, move it to the utility room, and check it every five minutes until the heart stops beating," the doctor orders over the telephone.

Marcy, seventeen years old, decided with great difficulty to go ahead with this abortion just recently, twenty weeks into an unwanted pregnancy. Usually, after several hours of hard labor caused by an injection of *prostaglandin,* the baby is stillborn, but Marcy has delivered a critically ill baby girl who weighs well under a pound.

The nurse wraps the child in a towel, cuts the umbilical cord, and heads for the utility room, agonizing over what she is about to do. "I can't do this!" she decides. "This baby is alive! I may get into serious trouble, but I must give her a chance." She contacts the pediatrician on call.

"I would really rather not get involved," the pediatrician answers. "The intent of the procedure was the death of the fetus. Besides, it can't possibly survive at this age and size. You can take it to the nursery if you want, but I will not come in to take care of it. Aggressive treatment is futile."

Gently the nurse places the newborn in a basinette, keeps her warm, tries to soothe her, and watches helplessly for an hour as she struggles to survive.

"Should I give her oxygen?" she questions. "Should I move her to an *Isolette* to give her added warmth? Should I fill out a birth certificate? Should I call the admitting office to obtain a hospital admission number for her? Should I start a chart to record my observations?"

After sixty-five minutes, the struggling stops; the child is dead. The nurse wonders, "Do we need to complete a death certificate? We would if the mother had wanted this child. In that case, everything possible would have been done to save her, and we all would have shared in the sorrow of her death."

THE HISTORY OF THE CONTROVERSY

What kind of societal ethic allows taking the lives of unborn babies in one room while encouraging the medical team next door to heroically save lives of babies the same size and age, when the only physical difference is that one is wanted and the other is not?

Both actions are *legal*. Is it possible that both are right?

Abortion, although widely practiced, was considered immoral and illegal in most modern western societies until this generation. The United States had many ethical rules against abortion, including state laws, hospital policies, and prohibitions in codes of medical practice. No one knows how many illegal abortions were done in this country, because the practitioners of illegal abortion kept no records. Techniques used were crude and dangerous, sometimes resulting in infection, sterility, or death.

The 1960s brought increasing activism in favor of legalizing abortion. Initially, the motives were to help women who were victims of rape or incest, and those who carried deformed babies, as well as to eliminate the dangers of illegal abortion. Later, the goal of the advocates became abortion-on-demand for any reason at all.

According to Bernard Nathanson, M.D. (an early leader in the National Abortion Rights League and a pioneer in legal abortion), pro-choice advocates began to garner sympathy for their cause by emphasizing (even exaggerating) the deaths of young women at the hands of back-street abortionists.[1] (Advances in fetal research subsequently convinced Dr. Nathanson that widespread abortion on demand was wrong, and he became an out-spoken protector of the unborn.)

Early Christian response to this pro-choice activism was mixed. Roman Catholics were consistent and steadfast in their opposition to abortion. Protestants were divided. Most liberal denominations were in favor of lessening restrictions on abortion and took strong pro-choice positions. Some have recently retreated somewhat and decry casual abortion; but most still believe it is a woman's right to choose to end an early unwanted pregnancy. Early in the debate, evangelicals tended to ignore the issue, fearing that it was part of the "social gospel" and would detract from their primary goal of sharing the gospel; most have subsequently adopted a pro-life position very close to that of the Catholics.

The U.S. Supreme Court's *Roe v. Wade* (see appendix) ruling in January of 1973 struck down all state laws that restricted abortion. It said that the states could not forbid or regulate abortions in the first third of pregnancy, but could pass laws that would regulate the procedure in the second third. In the final third of pregnancy, the ruling said the state's interest in the life of the unborn might allow it to pass laws to forbid abortion, but abortion could not be prohibited in circumstances where the life or health of the woman were at stake. The concept of health was broadly interpreted to mean that a perceived threat to the woman's mental well-being could justify an abortion. Since any unwanted pregnancy can induce considerable emotional turmoil, and since most pregnancies are detected before the third trimester, abortion-on-demand has become the practical outcome of *Roe v. Wade.*

MENTAL HEALTH

Jane pleaded for the life of the unborn baby. Eight weeks pregnant, her friend Susan had entered a psychiatric hospital, overcome with conflicting emotions. Susan had severe anxiety about trying to raise this child as a single parent. How foolish she had been to let her estranged husband visit that night and have sex with her! She knew that a reconciliation was not probable, considering his drinking and history of adultery.

Susan was already struggling to make ends meet for herself and her two other children. She told Jane that the doctors recommended an abortion for her mental health.

"That doesn't make it right," Jane argued. "There are other options, such as adoption." If she would only reconsider and give it a little more time.

Of the more than twenty million U.S. abortions performed since the 1973 Supreme Court decision, it is estimated that fewer than two percent have been done for the originally proposed reasons to justify abortion (i.e., rape, incest, or congenital malformations). In this same period, abortion techniques have become safer, so the 1960s argument for legalized abortion to prevent maternal injury and death is no longer significant. Thus, ninety-eight percent of currently performed abortions are done because the pregnancy is inconvenient.

POLARIZED POSITIONS

The controversy surrounding abortion is again increasing since the 1989 U.S. Supreme Court's *Webster v. Reproductive Services* decision allowing states to limit abortions in some cases (see appendix, for a discussion of this decision).

State elections are becoming pro-choice versus pro-life battle-grounds. There seems to be no middle ground. The polarization has come about in part because the opponents neither under-stand nor accept each other's logic and ethical priorities.

Pro-life advocates sometimes characterize their opponents as evil people whose goal is to make money by killing babies. Pro-choice advocates in turn characterize the pro-lifers as cold and unfeeling toward the woman experiencing an unwanted pregnancy. Most people on both sides have good intentions, but they put their emphasis on different ethical principles and use different methods of moral reasoning because they are operating under different world views.

How can honest people with good intentions reach such opposite conclusions about such an important issue?

THE RULES OF SOCIETIES CHANGE

Society's rules are not absolute; they change with time. That's what happened in 1973; all prior rules prohibiting abortion were deleted. The main reason for the change was a change in the prioritization of ethical principles that had occurred in the previous few years. For hundreds of years the value of the person ("sanctity of life") was considered more important than all other principles in medical ethics. When a conflict arose, the person's life was more important than truth, justice, self-determination, or any other principle.

For many, the value of human life was linked to a belief that each human being is created in the image of God (*imago dei*). The sanctity of life principle, however, was accepted and practiced by both believers and unbelievers.

In the 1960s, aware of the support for the sanctity of life principle, pro-choice advocates at first argued that life didn't begin at conception. Confronted with scientific facts that showed biological life does begin at conception, they later contended that "personhood" was separate and distinct from biological life, and was so ill-defined that society could not be rigid about the limits of its protection. Even more recently, they have conceded that potential human persons are sacrificed in the abortion process, but argue that the woman's *right to self-determination* is of greater ethical significance than *the value of the potential person.* Throughout the debate, pro-life advocates have maintained that in most cases the sanctity of life principle gives higher priority to the protection of the fetus than to the woman's freedom of choice. Pro-lifers have been accused of being indifferent to the woman's social concerns, condemning her to an unwanted pregnancy, and forcing her to bear a child who will be a burden.

MORAL REASONING HAS DECAYED

Until relatively recently in human history, moral reasoning has had these foundations:[2]

- There is a Creator-God.
- God has provided rules and principles regulating morality.
- Rightness and wrongness are measured by these standards.

Over the past few centuries, scientific endeavor has replaced God as the explainer of "mysteries," or source of truth, with the result that now many believe:

- There is no personal, supernatural God; therefore, *man* is sovereign (master of his own destiny).
- Man sets his own standards, which are relative.
- The morality of an act is determined by results, not rules.

In terms of ethics, personal self-determination (autonomy) has become more important than the sanctity of human life.

Therefore, the pro-life position needs other ways of explaining reality if it is to reach secular people in our "post-Christian" world. In other words, if the abortion debate is won by pro-lifers, it will be through a convincing appeal, in secular terms, focused on the status of the fetus in the context of the maternal-fetal environment.

Currently, five positions can be distinguished on this subject (percentages assigned are arbitrary):

MATERNAL RIGHTS VERSUS FETAL RIGHTS

Position	% Maternal rights	% Fetal rights	Comments
Total reproductive freedom	100	0	Abortion permissible at any time; fetus has no status.
Abortion-on-demand	70	30	Abortion permissible under most circumstances, but fetus has some status, depending on viability.
Balanced rights	30	70	Abortion problematic due to fetal status, but possible under some circumstances.
Right to life	2	98	Abortion very problematic, but okay in certain well-defined situations (rape, incest, actual threat to mother's life).
Absolute right to life	0	100	Abortion untenable under any circumstance; fetal surgery or C-section permissible even against mother's will, due to high fetal status.

The Case of the College Senior

As a result of "date rape," Ms. Wilson, a college senior, is eight weeks pregnant. She wishes to complete her education and would prefer to begin motherhood later when she's more prepared. The "father" is repentant and offers to marry Ms.

Wilson. She declines, stating that she certainly doesn't love him and that statistics indicate the marriage would almost certainly end in divorce. He urges her to continue the pregnancy. Ms. Wilson decides to seek advice, receiving these answers representing the five positions:

- *Total reproductive freedom.* "You can have an abortion, because you have a right to control what happens to your body."
- *Abortion-on-demand.* "Have an abortion if you want. The fetus is too small to survive anyway."
- *Balanced rights.* "A difficult decision; abortion is acceptable in this case, but you should seriously consider the child's rights, too."
- *Right to life.* "Although abortion can be permissible here because of the circumstances of conception, should the fetus be penalized (killed), when adoption would redeem some good from a bad situation?"
- *Absolute right to life.* "Abortion is never acceptable; it would be murdering an innocent victim whose life should always be protected."

Torn between these alternatives, Ms. Wilson is unable to make an immediate decision. However, after ten more weeks, during which she has consulted friends, family, medical, social, and finally spiritual counselors, she has reached a decision to terminate the pregnancy. Now she finds the two most lenient middle positions have changed, because the fetus may be *viable.*

The Fetus Is Alive

Bernard Nathanson, who resigned as director of the Center for Reproductive and Sexual Health in 1973 (the first and then largest abortion clinic in the western world), stated in the *New England Journal of Medicine* that he was deeply troubled by his "own increasing certainty that I had in fact presided over 60,000 deaths." He explains:

The Harvard criteria for the pronouncement of death asserts that if the subject is unresponsive to external stimuli (e.g., pain), if the deep reflexes are absent, if there are no spontaneous movements or respiratory efforts, if the *EEG* reveals no activity of the brain, one may conclude the patient is dead. If any or all of these criteria are absent, and the fetus does respond to pain, makes respiratory efforts, moves spontaneously, and has electroencephalographic activity—life must be present.[3]

THE FETUS AS A PERSON

Recent medical and legal developments make it more difficult to ignore the fetus as an individual, thus enhancing its status:

- the emergence of neonatal medicine which salvages critically ill, tiny premature newborns.
- the survival of fetuses after late abortions.
- ultrasound technology which enables mothers to see the human traits of the fetuses and perhaps even to "bond" with them.
- fetal surgery and other fetal therapy.
- the occupational protection of the fetus whose mother is now in the workplace.
- the growing recognition that passive smoking by the fetus is a form of child abuse.
- increasing public awareness of the impact on the fetus of alcohol or drug abuse by the mother, including conviction of a mother for "providing cocaine to another" because of its effects on her unborn baby.[4]

These recent developments all implicitly recognize fetal status. If these tiny individuals are patients who may be operated on, given medicine, protected from harmful environmental factors, and (very importantly) be easily seen through ultrasound, their rights as persons (even by secular, constitutional standards) cannot be as easily ignored.

THE BIBLE AND THE STATUS OF THE FETUS

While by themselves these arguments might be persuasive, for biblical Christians, the final word on the status of the fetus comes from Someone who understands the womb from outside and inside—having created us. The field narrows to Jesus, the only being who is like us but still other than us, One who lives and reigns with God and was God before the beginning of the world (John 1:1).

God's perspective as given to us in the Bible is able to tell us that which we can't know for sure on purely human terms: Is the living fetus "human"? Is the fetus an individual, loved by God? Is abortion really the taking of a separate human life? While some might argue that the Bible never discusses abortion, we have phrased the question carefully. The medical "procedure" of abortion is not the issue. Our concern is the status of the fetus, something the Bible does address in these following passages:

> For you created my inmost being; you knit me together in my mother's womb. I praise you because I am fearfully and wonderfully made; your works are wonderful, I know that full well. My frame was not hidden from you when I was made in the secret place. When I was woven together in the depths of the earth, your eyes saw my unformed body. All the days ordained for me were written in your book before one of them came to be. (Psalm 139:13-16)

> Before I was born the LORD called me; from my birth he has made mention of my name. . . . And now the LORD says—he who formed me in the womb to be his servant to bring Jacob back to him and gather Israel to himself. (Isaiah 49:1,5)

The word of the LORD came to me, saying, "Before I
formed you in the womb I knew you, before you were
born I set you apart; I appointed you as a prophet to the
nations." (Jeremiah 1:4-5)

These Old Testament passages, picked from many concerning the value of persons in the womb, illustrate God's
perception of the fetus. The unborn are formed by God's work-
manship and seen by Him; they are considered worthy to be
called by name; they are expected to be born and become shep-
herds, kings, and prophets. God is the maker of the unborn and
He seems to afford them the status of human beings (Job 3:3-4;
Psalm 95:6-7; 100:3; 119:73; Isaiah 44:2,24).

In the New Testament, Dr. Luke includes an intriguing
incident in his account of the events surrounding Jesus' birth.
Mary, only recently pregnant, visits Elizabeth, who is late in
her pregnancy with John. At the sound of Mary's greeting,
the pre-born John the Baptist leaps "for joy" within Elizabeth
(see Luke 1:41-45). This interesting interchange has several
implications for the status of the fetus:

- even before birth (in fact, indicated by the text, at least
  three months before birth), John was already fulfilling
  his prophetic role in relation to Jesus by confirming
  Mary's blessedness to Elizabeth, and he experienced
  joy in doing so;
- long before birth, perhaps only a few days or weeks
  after conception, Jesus was already a person worthy
  of honor.

Know Where You Stand, But Expect Others to Differ

Despite such a high view of the fetus in the Bible, Christians
have differed on the abortion issue for years, as they have on
many issues. One only needs to read the Christian literature to
see that this is the case. Some hold that abortion is never justified except to save the life of the mother, and the fetus should

be treated maximally even against the will of the mother. Others believe that this position devalues the status of the mother. Some would even say that Christian compassion for the mother justifies the agonizing decision for abortion in some difficult cases. A few argue that human personhood develops during gestation so that an early abortion is less evil than one done later in pregnancy. We believe that the Scriptural portrayal of the fetus is clear and thus abortion is rarely morally justified.

Regardless of the details of our beliefs about abortion, compassion is required of all who follow Christ. Rather than condemning the proponents of abortion, Christians need to respond in love. We should love others despite the choices they make. We should reach out to the woman with a crisis pregnancy, offering emotional, physical, financial, and spiritual assistance. Women confronting a crisis pregnancy often are facing the most difficult decision of their lives and recognize that they do not possess the strength or resources to carry on through the pregnancy.

Jesus taught not only compassion but social action as well (Matthew 25:31-46). This teaching should stimulate Christians to respect the beliefs of others even if they don't agree; to open their hearts, homes, and churches to love and help those who are in need. This compassionate outreach would seem to us to be more Christlike than the strident condemnation often heard from well-meaning protectors of the unborn.

Even when offered counsel and help, some women will find their circumstance so burdensome that they feel they cannot continue the pregnancy. Again, whether we personally believe their situation justifies their decision or not, we must continue to reach out to them in *agape* love, helping them experience God's grace and Christian fellowship.

Evangelicals need to understand the biblical principles and the ethical principles involved in the abortion debate; they need to be firmly convinced and committed to their position; they need to back up this position with support for the people involved, and to speak out in defense of both the woman and the fetus, who are intertwined. Some Christians will decide to become personally involved in trying to bring change through political action. Some will feel led to engage in forms of public protests or civil disobedience. Each should follow the example of Jesus, while always remembering that abortion is not, in the end, about issues, politics, or theology. It is about people.

AN EYE TOWARD THE FUTURE

Medically

The potential future legalization of the abortion pill, RU 486, will complicate the abortion controversy. RU 486 causes termination of pregnancy by inhibiting progesterone, which the body normally secretes after fertilization to prepare the uterine lining for implantation of the fertilized ovum. Since this pill can be taken at home, the nature of the debate will change, and the focus on abortion clinics may diminish.

If this pill becomes available, it will replace methods of contraception for many, since unwanted pregnancies become an easily solved, highly private problem. The pill will "discourage self-critical abortion decisions and reflection on the psychosocial relation of abortion to other forms of killing."[5]

The sexual partner will have even less reason for concern than he has now, and will almost surely not give pause to reflect on the actual consequences of his sexual activity.

Legally

Even if significant legal changes occur (i.e., changes in *Roe v. Wade*), abortion will remain a contentious and divisive issue which defies consensus. The rights of the woman will remain important, but there will be an increasing focus on the rights of the fetus. The environmental movement began in earnest after we saw NASA's stunning pictures of our fragile earth from space; in the same way a new appreciation for the tenuous life of the unborn is now possible with fetal photographs and ultrasounds. Consequently, more Americans will be increasingly open to a new consideration of the fetus as a visible human being. As we begin to see the fetus as God sees him or her—as our technology reveals the formerly secret process of being woven together in a wonderful fashion—we will better understand the need to love and cherish the unborn.

FOR DISCUSSION

Abortion is an emotionally charged discussion topic, for many reasons. During this session, you should keep in mind that someone in the room may have had an abortion or been involved with someone who had an abortion. On the other side, perhaps someone is present who has even been jailed (as in "Operation Rescue") in an effort to save endangered unborn lives. Also, men and women often have very different thoughts and feelings about this topic.

In your effort to speak the truth, remember that doing so in love requires compassion and understanding, and leaves no room for self-righteousness. Thoughtless words can wound a person you care about deeply.

Opening: To begin, have group members answer this question: Do you know someone personally who has had an abortion? How does knowing—or not knowing—someone personally affect your feelings and attitudes toward this issue?

1. Give each person who wishes a chance to answer this question: Where would you put yourself on the chart on page 53? What percent of rights do you think the fetus has? What percent do you think the mother has?

2. What reasons can you give to defend the idea that the fetus has rights? What reasons can be given to defend the mother's rights?

3. How would you counsel the college senior, Ms. Wilson (pages 53-54)? If you exhorted her to carry the baby to term, would you be willing to adopt it? Or, if her family should disown her for deciding to carry the baby to term, would you be willing to take her in? Why, or why not?

4. In the past, the two sons of your pastor and his wife were afflicted with a very rare genetic defect, causing one to die and leaving the other handicapped, although their daughters were not afflicted. Now, despite contraception, it has been confirmed that Mrs. Bates is pregnant, and through *amniocentesis* it is also confirmed that the fetus is male.

   As your pastor's best friend, who has shared the past years of agony and despair with him, you try to help him focus his thinking regarding this crisis, which occurs on several levels.
   a. What are these levels?
   b. What are Rev. and Mrs. Bates' options?
   c. What principles collide here, and which take precedence? What biblical passages would you bring to mind?
   d. How would you pray about this?
   e. Are you surprised when he comments that now, though he has been outspoken against abortion, he understands the other side better? Why, or why not?

5. As a family doctor, you make it your policy to ask adolescents in your care about their sexual activity. Within this context of trust, you have discovered that many Christian young people are sexually active. Now your friend's sixteen-year-old daughter has made an appointment with you, because she knows you have counseled one of her friends.

   Role-play the office conversation with her, with two volunteers in the group. Would you give her advice on contraception? Would you provide her with the birth control pill or condoms?

6. One of your friends, Becky, was recently imprisoned after an "Operation Rescue," and she is still incarcerated a week later because she will not give her real name.
   a. Your five-year-old daughter asks you what awful thing Becky has done. How do you respond?
   b. Your answer is so supportive that your daughter suggests, "Then why don't we go down into prison with her, Mommy, if we can keep some babies from being killed?" Now what will you say and do?
   c. Finally, Becky is released. But as you hear her talk about it, and especially as she refers to the apathy of the church you attend together, you think she's beginning to sound a little self-righteous. Then she announces she is going to participate in another rescue next week and invites you. How do you respond now?

APPENDIX: SUPREME COURT DECISIONS

Roe v. Wade and Doe v. Bolton

On January 22, 1973, the U.S. Supreme Court announced its findings in two controversial landmark cases, *Roe v. Wade* and a companion case, *Doe v. Bolton*. The Court decided:

1. In the first trimester, the decision regarding abortion should be between the woman and her physician.
2. In the second trimester, the state, in order to promote its interest in the health of the pregnant woman, may choose to regulate the abortion decision to protect maternal health.
3. After viability, the state can regulate and even prohibit abortion except where necessary for the preservation of the life or health of the pregnant woman.

Justice Blackmun delivered the opinion of the Court. An important quote from his opinion is as follows:

One reason for the adoption of criminal abortion laws
[like Texas' where the Roe case began] was the concern
with abortion as a medical procedure. When most [laws]
were first enacted, the procedure was a hazardous
one for the woman. [Modern] medical techniques have
altered this situation. [Medical data indicate] that abortion in early pregnancy, that is, prior to the end of the
first trimester, although not without its risk, is now relatively safe. [But] important state interests in the area of
health and medical standards do remain. The State has
a legitimate interest in seeing to it that abortion, like
any other medical procedure, is performed under circumstances that ensure maximum safety for the patient.
[The] State retains a definite interest in protecting the
woman's own health and safety when an abortion is proposed at a late stage of pregnancy.

[There is also] the State's interest [in] protecting
prenatal life. [Logically], of course, a legitimate state
interest in this area need not stand or fall on the acceptance of the belief that life begins at conception or at
some other point prior to live birth. In assessing the
State's interest, recognition may be given to the less
rigid claim that as long as potential life is involved,
the State may assert interests beyond the protection of
the pregnant woman alone. [It] is with these interests,
and the weight to be attached to them, that this case is
concerned.

The Court recognized that certain zones of privacy exist
under the constitution—marriage, procreation, contraception,
family relationships, child-rearing, and education.

All Christians with an active interest or involvement in
the abortion controversy should read *Roe v. Wade* (which is less
than one hundred pages long), so they can better understand
the current legal controversy over changes in this law—a controversy which began to heat up last year with *Webster*.

Webster v. Reproductive Health Services

In July 1989, the U.S. Supreme Court in *Webster v. Reproductive Health Services* upheld a Missouri law that prohibits abortions in public hospitals and in other taxpayer-supported institutions. There is disagreement among both pro-choice and pro-life forces about the future implications of the *Webster* ruling. Some think the Court will turn the clock back to pre-*Roe* days, while others think there will be little or no change in *Roe*. A few states have reacted to *Roe v. Wade* by new legislative activity that tends to restrict abortions. Examples of these restrictions include requiring parental consent in the abortion for a minor.

NOTES:
1. Bernard N. Nathanson, *Aborting America* (New York: Doubleday, 1975).
2. Francis A. Schaeffer and C. Everett Koop, *Whatever Happened to the Human Race?* (Old Tappan, NJ: Revell, 1979).
3. Bernard N. Nathanson, "Deeper into Abortion," *New England Journal of Medicine*, November 28, 1974, 291:1189.
4. Daniel Callahan, "How Technology Is Reframing the Abortion Debate," *Hastings Center Report*, February 1986, 16(1):33-42.
5. Lisa S. Cahill, " 'Abortion Pill' RU 486: Ethics, Rhetoric, and Social Practice," *Hastings Center Report*, October-November 1987, 17(5):5-8.

Chapter Four

The Dreaded Surprise

"What are you trying to save?" the pediatrician asked, looking over the Christian doctor's shoulder into the *Isolette*. "I don't know, Pete . . . but he's struggling to stay alive."

Joan and Murray had been hoping for a boy. They had two girls already, this child would be their last. Pregnancy and labor were normal, but as the head emerged it looked abnormally large and was not symmetrical. Delivery of the body revealed multiple structural defects. The baby was making no attempt to breathe, but did have a strong heartbeat and good muscle tone on one side of his body.

"It's a boy," the doctor said to the parents, quickly clamping and cutting the cord. "He has some problems and is having difficulty breathing. I need to take him to the nursery right away. I'll be back as soon as I can to let you know what is happening."

The baby was placed in a pre-warmed Isolette to receive

oxygen, and after a few puffs of artificial respiration, he started to make a few gasps and grunts, just as the pediatrician on call arrived.

A quick examination revealed that the left side of the boy's body seemed intact and normal. The right side of his head was smaller than the left. There was a marked curvature of the upper spine to the right so that the right side of the chest was very small. The right upper arm was absent, the elbow attached at the shoulder. The forearm was very short, and the fingers of the right hand were scrambled so that they pointed five different directions. The right hip was dislocated; the leg itself seemed normal except that the toes were also scrambled. A significant portion of the skin on the right side of the body was covered with what appeared to be irregularly shaped, thick, rough birthmarks.

Immediately, decisions had to be made.

How vigorous should be the resuscitation? Who should make that decision? Should the doctor make it alone? Should the pediatrician help? Is there time to call the *neonatal* specialists at the medical center? Should they ask the parents to participate? Is there time for them to consult with family, friends, clergy? Should the hospital ethics committee be involved? What is the prognosis? Are the baby's defects incompatible with life? Does he have abnormalities of internal organs as well? If so, will they affect his health and functioning? Will he be retarded? If so, how severely? Should these considerations impact the decision about resuscitation? (See case note 1, page 78, to see how this turned out.)

A "NORMAL" BABY?

"Will my baby be normal?" Most pregnant women ask this question. Some ask their husband, mother, or friends. Some ask their physician. Some ask God. For some, this question is so fearsome they are even afraid to ask themselves.

In the past the answer was, "Only God knows." Today,

better knowledge of genetics and the availability of *sonography* and *amniocentesis* have made it possible to detect some kinds of birth defects prior to delivery. But most abnormalities go undetected until birth or sometime later.

What is normal anyway? It is estimated that four percent of all newborns in the United States have some abnormality. Some of these are minor, such as a "birthmark" in a spot that will not be visible. Such things are considered "normal variants." Some abnormalities are significant but correctable, such as a cleft lip or club foot. Others are severe and may be life-threatening, such as *spina bifida* and severe heart defects. Newborns with these problems are critically ill and may not survive. In addition, babies born very prematurely and those who suffer severe injury or infection at the time of birth are also in danger of imminent death.

In the past, medical care for these critically ill newborns consisted mainly of maintaining warmth and nutrition. Survival was neither predictable nor controllable. However, advances in neonatal care in the past two or three decades have made it possible to sustain the lives of many of these imperiled newborns.

Some of their problems are correctable:

- with time (e.g., maturation of the lungs in the *preemie*);
- with medications (e.g., neonatal infections);
- with surgery (e.g., some heart defects).

Other problems are only partially correctable and leave a surviving infant with minor or major handicaps. Still others are not correctable at all, but the infant's life may be prolonged for a few weeks, months, or years.

Over the past fifteen years, there has been increasing controversy over appropriate treatment for these critically ill babies.[1] The debate includes physicians, ethicists, lawyers, parents, theologians, and spokespersons for the disabled.

Occasionally, specific cases are discussed in the popular

press as well. These articles often focus on dramatic cases—like a mentally retarded newborn who needs life-saving surgery to correct a fatal physical defect. Or an infant with a major birth defect who is expected to suffer physical and/or mental impairment even if operated on but who will have greater impairment or will die if surgery is withheld.

In the delivery room or nursery, the issues are often more diverse than the stories that make the newspapers. Some of these critical decisions must be made in a few moments, as with Joan and Murray's child. Other cases allow for a more reasoned approach.

A BROKEN HEART

Melissa was seventeen and unmarried when her pregnancy was confirmed. She and Chet decided on a hasty wedding and both their families were supportive. She dropped out of school; he found a steady job; they rented a mobile home. They struggled through this turmoil of sudden changes, and eventually life began to settle down to near normal. Melissa was about two months away from her due date when the bad news came.

Dr. Nelson thought that Melissa's baby was growing a little more slowly than average. During one prenatal visit, the doctor also noticed that the baby's heartbeat was very irregular. She ordered a sonogram and the result was bizarre. The baby seemed to be a little small, but was normally formed except for one severe defect. Its heart was located on the outside of the chest, and the heart itself was abnormally formed. Both of the parents were distraught when they were told the news. They spent a long time that day and again two days later discussing treatment options with Dr. Nelson.

Should they proceed with the planned vaginal delivery at their community hospital? If so, should the neonatal transport team from the medical center be present at the time of delivery to take the baby to the Neonatal Intensive Care Unit (NICU)? Because of the possibility that the heart might be compressed during delivery enough to kill the baby, should Dr. Nelson plan to do a Cesarean section when Melissa went into labor? Should her obstetrical care be transferred to a large teaching hospital two hours away so that she could deliver near the NICU? If the baby survived delivery, should he or she undergo surgery to have the heart placed in the chest cavity?

The pivotal question in making these decisions was the *prognosis*. Dr. Nelson had done her homework. She had consulted textbooks and recent journal articles and had called neonatologists at two respected medical centers. None of these sources were encouraging. Of the forty-three cases of this condition (*ectopia cordis*) reported in the literature, forty had severe heart defects and all had died with or without surgical correction. The three whose hearts were normal (other than being outside their bodies) had survived for over a year after surgery, but had been very ill throughout their short lives.

The neonatologist at the medical center said that if the baby were delivered there, he would feel obligated to do surgery. He said it was a teaching institution, and although they suspected the baby would not survive, it would give them more surgical experience so that a future patient with a normal heart would have a better chance of survival.

After several days of thought, tears, confusion, and discussion, Melissa and Chet told Dr. Nelson that they had decided to proceed with vaginal delivery at the community hospital. If the baby survived birth, they wanted to keep it with them, give it comfort and support and nourishment, but not have it subjected to the pain of futile surgery.

This decision settled the question for the parents, but now Dr. Nelson faced a new set of questions: Was the parents' decision in the baby's best interests? Should she ask for an ethics committee consultation? Should she ask any social or legal agency to get involved? (See case note 2 to discover the outcome of this case.)

Because a handicapped newborn cannot speak or decide, someone else—a *surrogate*—must decide for him. Will he live or die? If he lives, how impaired will he be? Who decides, and how?

What is ethically correct for a particularly handicapped newborn?

What factors should be considered? What roles do the different people play? How do their varying perspectives influence their decision?

THE IMAGE OF GOD

Scripture speaks of man being made in the image of God (Genesis 1:26-27, 5:1; 1 Corinthians 11:7). This Judeo-Christian tradition of the imago dei is the basis for personhood, dignity, and basic human rights. This biblical concept of the person affirms that each infant born possesses an intrinsic dignity which entitles him to receive whatever medical care is thought to be in his or her best interests.

It may seem absurd to say that a grossly deformed or severely retarded newborn represents the image of God. After all, God is perfect and these babies are not. By this definition, however, we are all "rejects." Very few of us are totally satisfied with our bodies and minds. Thus, "defects" are matters of degree and perspective. We do not mean to say that some birth defects are not overwhelming. But in many cases, the question is one of perception.

For instance, one very famous weight lifter complained about his body's lack of "perfection." Similarly, a model whose face was internationally acclaimed as beautiful stated that she did not consider herself beautiful. Evidently, in both of these cases, the individual's ideal of perfection was not achieved.

The perfection we recognize in God is not a physical perfection. We don't even know if God has a "body." We know Him as spirit. The image of God in man is a spiritual reality. The human spirit is like Him in some way and is capable of perfection as the result of regeneration (Romans 8:29, Colossians 3:10).

Parents of handicapped children often ask, "Why did God do this? Why did He allow this to happen?" The "why" questions are often the hardest to answer.

God claims His sovereignty, even in relation to handicaps. When Moses complained that he was "slow of speech and tongue," God responded by saying, "Who gave man his mouth? Who makes him deaf or mute? Who gives him sight or makes him blind? Is it not I, the LORD? Now go; I will help you speak and will teach you what to say" (Exodus 4:11). Not only does God affirm His involvement here, He teaches us to rely on Him for help and direction in these difficult situations. When we are inclined to ask "why?" we should instead ask "how?" and know that He is there to answer.

If we conclude that, in the eyes of God, all newborns are of equal worth, why must non-treatment decisions be made? Why not just treat all newborns with all means available? This simplistic approach to medical ethics is very attractive at first glance, because it makes it unnecessary to struggle with difficult decisions. But just because technology says, "We can do it!" does not mean "We should do it." There are some situations where aggressive treatment may be ethically foregone, and there are even some situations where aggressive treatment may be wrong because it prolongs the suffering of a dying newborn.[2] Someone must discern; someone must decide.

WHO WILL DECIDE?

Under normal circumstances, with a healthy newborn, parents make the decisions impacting the child. Will the infant be fed by breast or bottle? Will solid foods be given early or late? Will a son be circumcised? Will children be immunized? What about fluoride? They may seek advice from parents, friends, books, or medical professionals, but even when things are "normal," parents face a multitude of treatment decisions.

When their newborn is handicapped, the parents are the morally and legally recognized surrogates for the child. They must decide, sometimes weighing very difficult alternatives which may not have a clearly defined right or wrong answer. If time allows, after talking with the pediatrician, they may choose to consult with family members, spiritual advisers, ethics consultants or committees, or the families of other handicapped children before making a treatment or nontreatment decision.

The Doctor's Role

The primary role of the attending physician is that of advocate for the patient. Have all reasonable medical measures been taken in the best interests of the infant? A secondary role is that of medical consultant for the parents. The doctor must thoroughly assess and confirm the diagnosis and prognosis of the infant and communicate this information to the family in a fashion they can understand. The doctor must counsel the parents and provide access to others who may help them reach a decision. Parents also need adequate time and an appropriate environment to reach a thoughtful decision.

The physician must be as objective as possible in regard to the prognosis, giving hard data instead of generalizations. Telling the parents of a baby with *Down syndrome* that the child will be "a blob," as one physician recently did, is not only misleading but factually inaccurate. But even if a physician's facts are correct, there is no way to totally eliminate the impact of the doctor's bias. The parents will likely request an opinion on what should be done, or what the physician would do if this were his own child. The doctor may offer his ethical opinion as well as what he believes to be the consensus among other physicians and ethicists. This is the physician's job, but parents must understand that they are free to disagree.

Making recommendations is part of the physician's role, but he or she may fail in that role in two very different ways. The doctor may hide behind the "objectivity" of the medical facts and refuse to give any guidance on what is medically or ethically correct, merely saying "These are the options. What do you want to do?" Conversely, the physician may coerce the parents into making a decision that she prefers by relating only those facts that will produce that decision. As she walks this very fine line, she should try to point out to the parents when she is giving medical facts and when she is offering ethical opinion. She must also encourage the parents to get second and third opinions. If the ethical issues are not clear to her or to the parents, the doctor should suggest a consultation with the ethics committee (if the hospital has one). Some hospitals have special committees set up just to review situations involving imperiled newborns. Names of two such committees are Infant Care Review Committee and Infant Bioethics Committee.

Sometimes Others Must Intervene
In rare cases, the responsibility for a treatment decision is taken from the parents, perhaps due to mental impairment or because the emotional trauma of the situation has rendered them unable to decide. Occasionally parents will have an unresolvable disagreement about what to do. Once in a while, the parents make a decision that is clearly not in the infant's best interests. It is at these times that the physician's role as advocate for the infant becomes critical. He must do his best to resolve the situation in the best interests of the infant, and if necessary he should petition the probate court for appointment of a legal guardian and request judicial review of the decision.

WHAT IS RIGHT, WHAT IS WRONG?

Sometimes the decision whether to treat a particular birth defect is easy. For example, occasionally a baby is born with incomplete development of the *esophagus* so that food is unable to pass from the mouth to the stomach. This condition is called *esophageal atresia*. Without corrective surgery, the baby will be unable to eat and will die. Major surgery soon after birth gives good results. There is no question that the surgery should be done. If for some unexplainable reason the parents refuse to give consent for the procedure, the physicians involved ought to petition the court for judicial intervention on behalf of the infant.

Decisions may not seem quite as straightforward if the baby with esophageal atresia is also afflicted with Down syndrome. There are some who believe that surgical correction of the obstruction in this situation is optional and should not be done if the parents wish to let the baby die. Such was the situation in the Bloomington, Indiana, *Baby Doe* case in 1982. After discussing the prognosis for Down syndrome (and being told by one physician that the baby would be a "blob"), the parents chose to decline surgery. This was challenged in a local court, but the court upheld the parents' right to refuse surgery, and the baby was allowed to die.

The *Baby Doe* case has been the subject of much legal and ethical debate. On review, it appears that the parents were given an unusually pessimistic picture of the future for their child. One of the physicians involved gave a biased prognosis and thus influenced the parents so that they chose a course of non-treatment that suited the physician's utilitarian ethic. The decision against surgery was based not on the outcome of surgery, but on the inappropriate prognosis and bias of the physician. Most physicians, lawyers, and ethicists agree that this decision was ethically incorrect, and most practicing pediatricians would treat "Baby Doe."[3] As a result of this case, the federal government promulgated the controversial *Baby Doe* regulations, which attempt to influence the circumstances where treatment of handicapped newborns may be limited.

There Is Room for Debate

The picture becomes more clouded in cases where aggressive treatment gives only a small chance of survival, or where that survival will include major handicaps with great suffering for the patient and a significant burden—financial or otherwise—for the family or society. In such cases, there is no simple formula that produces dogmatic yes or no decisions. There is room for disagreement among Christians and even among family members.

When a treatment versus a non-treatment decision must be made quickly, and the prognosis is not clearly hopeless—as with Joan and Murray's newborn son—it is ethically imperative to choose treatment. Choosing non-treatment in such a circumstance is an irreversible decision. After treatment is started, if it becomes apparent that the outlook is truly hopeless, it is ethically permissible to discontinue the treatment.

In those rare instances where a choice is made for less than maximal treatment, the responsibility for nurturing remains. The infant should still be comforted, kept warm, offered food and should be treated for pain. This seems humane and obvious and should always be done. For example, if a baby is born very prematurely so that there is no precedent for survival, then it is not ethically required to transfer the child to the Neonatal Intensive Care Unit, use a respirator, or otherwise provide extraordinary care. However, the infant should always receive appropriate holding, nurturing, and feeding.

Balancing "Best Interests"

One of the most difficult aspects of decision-making regarding handicapped newborns is knowing what is in "the best interests of the infant." This phrase is subjective and value-laden. Is it ever in one's best interest to die? Consider how difficult it sometimes is for an adult to decide what is in his own best interest:

- Should I have this risky surgery to unplug a blocked artery in my neck?
- Should I undergo chemotherapy, which will not cure

my cancer but may prolong my life a few months, while making me feel sick in the process?

How much more difficult it is to make comparable decisions for infants whom God has entrusted to our care. Is it ever in the best interest of the child to decline life-saving surgery that will leave him severely disabled? If the infant were able to speak, would he or she ever choose death over life with a severe handicap? Should the pain and expense of the proposed treatment be a consideration? What about the physical, emotional and financial burden imposed on the family?

While this burden may be substantial, it is important to note that C. Everett Koop, M.D., former Pediatric Surgeon in Chief at Philadelphia Childrens Hospital and U.S. Surgeon General, states that no patient or family under his care has ever retrospectively questioned the wisdom of doing heroic surgery on a handicapped newborn, even when the resulting life was severely handicapped. The consensus was that life is worth living.[4]

The burden a severely disabled child places on his or her family is difficult to assess, and such calculations can lead to a utilitarian ethic. In its most extreme view, utilitarianism allows some individuals, even groups of individuals, to be eradicated because they are or may become a burden on society—physically, emotionally, financially. The old . . . the unborn . . . the handicapped . . . the intellectually inferior . . . ethnic groups . . . anyone who creates inconvenience or burden is at risk. Followed to its logical conclusion, the entire spectrum of human beings is at risk, subject to the changing definitions of those in power.

THE "LEAST OF THESE"

The "argument of burden" fails to consider the significant value to the family, and to society as a collection of families, that handicapped and disabled persons can bring into our shared experience as human beings. Without glorifying the tragedy of disabled children, we need to recognize that:

- Through them, we can learn to give and receive love in totally new ways.
- Through them, we can learn to appreciate as gifts some things we might otherwise take for granted: the ability to move about at will, to plan and carry out our dreams, to think clearly, to produce income, to become independent, to marry and to have a family, to grow old and retire to a place of our own choosing.
- Through them, we can learn to see richer hues in such deeper things as trust, simplicity, and joy.
- Through them, we can learn lessons of patience, courage, values, beauty, and true character. Without them, we who are cursed with normalcy might never know.

Such lessons cannot be bought at any price, nor can they be learned through lectures, books, or observation. They must be lived. It is through the pain of struggling with limitations—call them handicaps—in ourselves or those we love, that we more clearly see a fact of our existence that opens the way toward wisdom and knowing we are totally dependent upon our Creator.

Quality of Life Is Much Broader Than Utility

At least in some cases, a family's quality of life can be greatly *enhanced* through the presence of a handicapped child. One physician, Dr. Tom Elkins, wrote this moving tribute to his daughter, a child with Down syndrome:

To those Baby Does within our society, I would like to close with a message of thanks. These comments will sound strange to some who see abnormalcy as being unacceptable, because they speak about the Baby Does

in terms of the burdens imposed, with no attention to
the benefits provided as a result of treatment, or to
the quality of life someone anticipates they may one
day have. We counter their worthy debate, not with
columns of data and financial logic, but with joyful
experiences with our own child. We remember her wide
eyes and stretched grin as she tore into her birthday
packages, holding each item high and screaming "YEA!"
We remember a lunch table set perfectly and a little
girl with a perked smile gleaming at us with hands
folded under her chin. We remember her laughter as
she sat cross-legged while the family puppy leaped all
over her and licked her face. For giving new importance to the term "joy" in our home, we say thank you.
We also say thank you for your determination to perform the menial accomplishments of life that we take
for granted.

In our ingratitude we recognize the fallacy of our
pride and realize the peace that humility brings. You
become only an image of the self we each might be. That
self is frightening because we see our fragile normalcy
and our stark limitedness. But it is nonetheless the
humanity we share. For our humanity is entangled
with suffering experiences which we could dismiss
as meaningless, were it not for the demands that you
make on us to be loving. In those demands we finally
begin to understand the concept of costly, agonizing
grace. In a world so oriented to success and rewards,
you teach us to love without measuring what we gain
by loving. Thank you.[5]

CASE NOTES

Case Note 1: Joan and Murray's baby boy responded well to
resuscitation and didn't seem to have any serious internal
abnormalities. He grew slowly, but developed well. Over the

next several years he had multiple orthopedic and plastic surgical procedures. He is well-integrated into their active family and is intellectually precocious.

Case Note 2: Chet and Melissa's baby survived birth. With help from the nurses, they lovingly provided tender care, and the baby died in his mother's arms of heart failure at three days of age.

FOR DISCUSSION

Opening: Give everyone in the group one minute to sketch out his or her personal experience with handicapped newborns.

1. Suppose you were Joan or Murray, the parents of the multiply handicapped newborn discussed on pages 65-66.
   a. Would you want the doctor to try to save the baby's life?
   b. If you knew that for every day in the hospital there would be four hundred dollars due after your insurance paid their part, would this affect your decision?
   c. On what basis might you decide that additional intervention would be futile?
   d. Who would you involve in helping you reach this decision?

2. Is it absurd to say that a grossly deformed or retarded newborn represents the image of God? In what sense can this be true, and where would you draw the yes/no line in relation to treatment for children with severe handicaps or birth aberrations?

3. Why not simply treat all newborns with all means available? Give scriptural as well as other dimensions of an answer.

4. While on a missions trip—as a helper in a local clinic—you are present for the birth of a child with hydrocephalus

(excess cerebrospinal fluid usually causing enlargement of the skull and atrophy of the brain). Although the hydrocephalus could be treated in the United States, in this remote village the child is simply left to die. When you express your dismay, you are told, "In this country, this is best. It is the will of God. The mother is young. She will have many more children."

After returning home, how might this experience affect your perspective on the question of handicapped newborns?

5. At what point, if any, would an infant's quality of life be so poor that nontreatment would be appropriate? Would permanent coma fit in this category?

6. *On your own:* Interview someone with a handicapped child, asking at least these questions: Has anything positive come from your experience? If so, what? If you could have known all the negatives in advance, what would you have done differently?

Report to your group what you learn.

NOTES:
1. Raymond S. Duff and A. G. M. Campbell, "Moral and Ethical Dilemmas in a Special Care Nursery," *New England Journal of Medicine,* October 25, 1973, page 890.
2. John D. Lantos, Steven H. Miles, Marc D. Silverstein, and Carol B. Stocking, "Survival After Cardiopulmonary Resuscitation in Babies of Very Low Birthweight: Is CPR Futile Therapy?" *New England Journal of Medicine,* January 14, 1988, 318:91-95.
3. I. David Todres, Jeanne Guillemin, and Michael A. Grodin, "Life-Saving Therapy for Newborns: A Questionnaire Survey in the State of Massachusetts," *Pediatrics,* May 1988, 81:643-649.
4. Francis A. Schaeffer and C. Everett Koop, *Whatever Happened to the Human Race?* (Old Tappan, NJ: Revell, 1979).
5. Tom Elkins and Douglas Brown, "Baby Doe and the Concept of Grace," *Christian Medical Dental Society Journal,* Spring 1987, 18(3):5-9; from the book *Faith for Troubled Times: Encouragement for Sufferers and Servants in Health Care* (Nashville, TN: Broadman Books, n.d.).

Chapter Five

What Would John Want?

After all we've been through, Norman thought, *how can John die now from a runny nose?*

It was so hard to concentrate . . . to understand . . . to comprehend the significance of what the doctor was saying.

"But . . . how can that be?" Norman protested. "It's just a runny nose. People don't die from runny noses."

"It is complicated . . . ," Dr. Whitney continued. But Norman's mind drifted. Just another complication, the latest in a series of crises that had begun fourteen months earlier.

His mind returned again to that 2:00 a.m. phone call, yanking him and Maria from a sound sleep into stark fear, followed by what would seem an endless night. Even now he felt a surge of adrenalin, a wave of raw emotion as he relived that frozen moment: "Hello . . . this is the emergency room . . . there's been an accident . . . your son . . . critical condition . . . truck . . . stone wall . . . can you come down right away?"

Hours stretched into days and days into weeks, as the focus of their entire lives became that hospital, that medical team, and most of all their twenty-five-year-old's struggle to live.

Now it was mostly a vague recollection, movements and repetitions, like some horrific drama with them both audience and cast, gliding to and fro through shadows and mist:

Head injury, coma, x-rays, waiting;

Multiple fractures, ventilator, coffee;

Depressed skull fracture, tears, surgery, hope, waiting;

I.C.U., prayer, family, phone calls, fear;

Waiting, waiting, waiting.

It seemed like only yesterday, and yet it seemed like forever.

IMPOSSIBLE CHOICES

The neurologist continued, "It seems that at the time of John's skull fracture, there was a small crack in the base of the skull that has never healed. It has allowed fluid from around his brain to leak into the tissues, and it has slowly tracked downward and now has appeared as a leak into the upper part of his nose. This is life-threatening, because it allows bacteria that live in the nose to move up and cause infection around the brain. This *meningitis* is treatable with antibiotics, but as long as that fluid leak persists, the infection will recur, and eventually the bacteria will develop resistance to antibiotics and take his life."

"It is possible," he continued, "to attempt surgical closure of the leak, but the surgery is both difficult and dangerous because it might cause further brain damage. We started treatment for the meningitis this morning, but we would like you two to decide which of three courses you would like us to take.

"One, attempt surgical correction of the leak which, if successful, would prevent further infection and allow him to live in his present condition, probably for many years.

"Two, use repeated antibiotics until they no longer work, in which case he would probably die in a few weeks.

"Or, three, stop antibiotics now, knowing that he will die in two or three days."

TIMING SOMEONE'S DEATH

"Dear God," Norman thought, "how can this be? How can it be that we have the authority to decide when our twenty-five-year-old son will die? We don't want to be in that position. What should we do? What do we want for John? What would he want for himself?"

Again he drifted back over the emotional roller-coaster months since the accident. In the beginning, they had seized every shred of hope: John's eyelids fluttered; he spent two hours off the ventilator today; did he grip Mom's hand when she touched his palm? But sometimes there was concern: He has a fever today; he's losing weight; he has pneumonia again.

After several months, John had been weaned off the ventilator, his weight was stabilized by tube feedings, and he was pronounced ready to leave the hospital to go to a chronic care facility. Was this a good omen? Or did this mean that the doctors thought he wasn't going to get much better and would be in the nursing home forever?

One year after the accident, his condition had a new label: *"persistent vegetative state"* (PVS). According to the neurologist, John remained unconscious, but not in a coma. He would be awake part of the time and asleep part of the time. Sometimes he would open his eyes, and they would wander without focusing on anything. He seemed unaware of his surroundings. He seemed unaware even of his parents.

Awake, but unaware. "Why, God?" Norman cried out within his soul. "Will this go on forever? How long is forever, God?"

WHO DECIDES, AND HOW?

Medical care involves decisions. Some cases are clear and require little or no discussion. Others are more complex and need a lot of thought and discussion. In recent years, diagnostic and therapeutic options have multiplied so dramatically that there are many more decisions that must be made. Sometimes the treatment options or the anticipated outcomes are so diverse, or so unpredictable, that a rational decision seems impossible.

Who makes the decision—the doctor, the patient, someone else? What if the patient is too young or too sick to participate in the decision? What if the patient is unable to speak, but has previously had very strong opinions about what should be done in such a circumstance? What if the patient is unable to speak, but has not given any indication what his or her opinion might be? What if there is major disagreement between interested parties (patient, physician, family members, etc); then who decides, and how?

Even Simple Cases Mean Choices

Little six-year-old Billy has had a fever and sore throat for three days. His mother decides to take him to the doctor since his throat is red and swollen with white spots, suggesting a possible strep infection.

The doctor decides a throat culture will be necessary, but the boy refuses to open his mouth to have it done.

- Does the doctor try to coerce the child into cooperation or proceed to forcefully do the culture?
- Does the doctor decide to treat for strep without doing the culture?
- Does the doctor ask the mother's opinion or permission?
- If a culture is done, does the physician start treatment with penicillin today or wait until tomorrow for the culture report?

- If the doctor decides to treat now, or if the culture is positive tomorrow, does he or she treat with penicillin by mouth or by injection?
- What if the boy refuses an injection?
- Once treatment is underway, does the doctor ask other family members to come in for cultures? Should the mother be asked to bring the boy back after treatment for a follow-up culture? And if the original culture is negative, does the doctor ask for a blood test for infectious mononucleosis? If so, when should the test be done?

Many decisions need to be made about Billy's simple medical problem. Some of these are so straightforward and risk-free that we don't even think of them as decisions; we just make them automatically without discussing other options.

For example, a positive throat culture for strep is automatically treated with penicillin in some form. (Unless, of course, the patient is allergic to penicillin; nothing is truly automatic in medicine!) Whether to use two-hundred-fifty milligrams four times a day or five-hundred milligrams twice a day by mouth; whether to use oral liquid or tablets; or whether to use one dose of long-acting injectable penicillin—these are minor decisions, but decisions that nonetheless have to be made.

Some of the decisions are not as clear-cut. For example, forcing an uncooperative child into some diagnostic or therapeutic procedure should not be done without careful consideration. Whether to treat today or wait for the culture requires balancing the cost of a prescription that might be wasted if the culture is negative versus the advantage of helping the child become well twenty-four hours sooner if the assumption is right.

Once the mother has made the decision to seek medical care for her son's sore throat, she usually expects the doctor to make most of these multiple decisions about diagnosis and treatment. Most of the decisions are easy, and the alternatives are almost risk-free. But they're not entirely without risk, of course. Untreated, strep can, on rare occasions, lead to rheumatic fever which can cause heart damage. Sometimes penicillin can cause a fatal reaction, especially when given by injection, and even very rarely when given by mouth. Such seemingly minor decisions may affect this child's health and maybe even his life. Decisions, decisions, decisions—about the management of Billy's sore throat!

THE CHANGING HORIZONS IN MEDICAL DECISION-MAKING

Until recent decades, most medical treatment decisions were made by the physician, based on what he or she felt was best for the patient. It was common for the doctor to withhold information or to pursue some treatment without taking the time to inform patients or involve them in the decision-making process.[1]

Sometimes family members also were involved in a web of deception:

"Is it cancer?" Fred whispered, almost choking on the word. He looked lovingly at his grandfather, who had emerged from surgery only hours earlier and was not yet fully conscious.

"Yes," his mother said quietly, tears streaming down her cheeks. "They couldn't get at it . . . gone too far."

"Can't anything be done?" Fred asked sadly.

"Just try to make him comfortable. A little more happiness."

"How long?"

"Six months, maybe eight."

"Do you think he knows?"

"Maybe . . . probably . . . he's seen it happen to others. But let's not tell him. Why depress him, after all, when nothing can be done about it? Besides, I don't think I can face talking about or even thinking about it myself . . . after the way Grandma died."

Recently, a major shift has taken place. The shift is away

from this paternalistic approach toward patient autonomy (patient rights). This is the end result of a gradual change in the patient-doctor relationship that has occurred over the past several generations. The "physician-priest" of ancient times was given nearly divine authority. The "physician-scientist" who emerged in the last century was held in awe for his technical knowledge and skills. The "physician-provider" of the last twenty years has been placed in a parsimonious contractual relationship with the "patient-consumer."[2] Final authority has shifted from physician to patient—or perhaps even from physician to patient to insurance companies.

INFORMED CONSENT

Informed consent is the central idea of patient-centered decision-making. This concept has emerged slowly over the past seventy years and means that a physician can't do anything to or for a patient without that patient's permission. Consent may be omitted when a true life-threatening emergency occurs that doesn't allow time to discuss the options. Consent is also unnecessary when the procedure is very simple and the risk very small.

The amount of detail required in the consent process depends on the risks involved, their likelihood, and their possible severity. For instance, if the patient runs a one in fifty risk of developing a rash from a medication that will be used in coronary artery surgery, and the rash is only a minor nuisance, it might not be mentioned in the consent process. However, if the patient runs a one in five hundred risk of death or serious disability from a particular aspect of the surgery, that definitely should be mentioned.

Consent is really a process of communication between patient and doctor. In order for the consent to be valid, the physician must give the patient adequate information, the patient must not be coerced, and the patient must be competent to give consent.

The Physician Must Give the Patient Adequate Information
A properly informed patient:

- Understands the procedure and the reason for doing it.
- Understands any significant risks and complications.
- Anticipates certain reasonable results.
- Knows about alternative procedures and the effects of not having a procedure done.
- Has received answers to all of his or her questions.

The Patient Must Not Be Coerced
"Your leg is getting worse, Nelly," Dr. Bishop said as gently as he could. His eighty-seven-year-old patient reminded him so much of his own mother.

"I know, Doctor," she answered. "It's my sugar."

"I'm afraid we need to operate," the doctor continued, watching Nelly's reactions carefully.

Slowly, she shook her head. Quietly she said, "No . . . not again."

Just three years earlier, Dr. Bishop had amputated Nelly's right leg. Now, in order to save her life, the gangrenous left leg would also need to be amputated.

"But, Nelly," he tried to reason with her. "If we don't do it, you could die from the infection."

"I know, Doctor. . . . I've lived long enough."

How could he convince her? She had a right to refuse, and she clearly understood the consequences. But how could he allow her to die when the surgery could give her another few years?

Dr. Bishop believed that the amputation was in Nelly's best interest, but he knew she did not want to have it done. He weighed his options:

- He might say, "If you don't have this done, you'll have to find yourself another doctor. You've just got to have this surgery. You'll die without it. You've got to sign for the surgery. I can't just stand idly by and watch you die when I've been trained to help." But this would be coercion.

• He might be tempted to manipulate her by exaggerating the benefits or understating the risks, but not only would that be unethical, it would be useless, since Nelly already knew what to expect.

So he wondered, is she competent? Do I need to involve someone else here? In the past, if the patient didn't agree with the doctor's recommendation, he or she was automatically considered incompetent. Because the patient didn't recognize the "infallible" wisdom of the doctor, his or her wishes were ignored.

The Patient Must Be Competent to Give Consent

In order to give valid consent, the patient must know what is going on. He or she does not have to be competent in the "global" sense—i.e., be able to balance a checkbook—in order to make medical decisions. But the patient does need to understand the information given, the decision that needs to be made, and the consequences of each decision option.

Most people you interact with daily meet this definition of competence. Not everyone does, however. Some mentally retarded people are capable of much independence, but are not capable of deciding whether to give consent for a kidney transplant. People who are under anesthesia, in a coma, or under the influence of drugs, alcohol, or medication may not be competent to make medical decisions. Likewise, those who are confused by mental illness or Alzheimer's may not have decision-making capacity.

By legal definition, minors (under the age of eighteen in most states) are not competent to make major health care decisions. In actuality, most adolescents should enter into the decision-making process with their parents. Many states give minors limited autonomy in that they are specifically allowed to obtain contraception, abortion, and treatment for venereal disease or substance abuse without parental permission.

Lack of decision-making capacity may be permanent, as for those with mental retardation or severe Alzheimer's disease; it may be temporary, as for the anesthetized patient; or it may vary from day to day, or even from hour to hour, as for some confused elderly people.

Although Nelly is elderly, she is not confused. She knows who she is, where she is, what day it is, and what is happening. Hers is a deliberate, measured choice, which is hers to make even if it will hasten her death.

OTHER DECISION-MAKERS

In some cases patients are not competent to make decisions. When this is true, someone else—a surrogate or substitute—must help. And sometimes this substitute decision-maker is brought in at the doctor's request.[3]

When a surrogate is asked to act for an incompetent patient, he or she must use one of two methods in reaching a decision. "Substituted judgment" is the guideline the surrogate uses if the patient has expressed a preference before becoming incompetent, or if the surrogate knows the patient well enough to know for sure what he or she would choose if still competent. In this case, the surrogate chooses what the patient would choose. When a surrogate has no clear idea what the patient would choose, he or she must use the more difficult method of "best interests": a method based on what is judged to be ultimately best for the patient.[4]

Dr. Bishop was unsettled. He knew an amputation would prolong Nelly's life. He knew she fully understood she would die if she refused surgery. He knew he could not ethically coerce her into the decision he would choose for her. He knew the patient's choice was supposed to supersede what might seem medically best. He didn't know whether the prospect of being a double amputee had made her so depressed that she was not thinking clearly. Had depression rendered her incompetent? If so, did she need a surrogate to make her decision for her?

After some thought, Dr. Bishop telephoned Nelly's son, Robert, who lived nearby, asking his assessment.

"I understand your reluctance to operate against her will, Doctor," he replied, "and I know Mother is adamant. All of us kids who live locally have discussed it, and none of us agrees with her. We've even told her how we love her and would like her to stay around awhile longer, but she just isn't about to change her mind. You know how she can be!"

Dr. Bishop hesitated, then asked, "Shall we get the court involved and ask that you or one of the other children be appointed her legal guardian?"

The conversation was silent for a long time as Nelly's son thought it through. Finally he answered, "Let me put it this way, Doctor. If it were me in her place, I think I would have the surgery. But if I had to make the decision for her, I would try to choose what she would choose, and we already know what she would do. She's told us. Hard as it is for all of us to let her have her way, I think it would do more harm than good to force her to lose the other leg. It would just hurt her and make her more depressed. It seems that this way she's planning to leave us on her terms and nobody else's."

Dr. Bishop became even more unsettled after a late-night call from Nelly's oldest son, the one living in Europe. Although this son, Jim, was almost never mentioned by the other siblings, Nelly had his picture in a prominent place on her dresser in the nursing home.

"Dr. Bishop," Jim began tentatively, "it's my understanding that Mother needs another amputation because of the infection in her leg."

"Yes," the doctor replied, "and without it, she will probably die. But," he continued, "your mother refuses to let me operate, and the other children seem resigned to letting her risk her life, when she could live several more years if we go ahead."

"I don't agree with the other children, Doctor . . . and, though they don't know it yet, I'm the executor of the estate. Mother trusts me. To be blunt, I think they would be relieved at her death, for several reasons: (1) They would no longer have the inconvenience of having to visit her; (2) there would no longer be the financial draw on the estate for the nursing home costs; and (3) they would finally have access to the considerable estate that my father left in trust."

"What would you suggest, then?" the doctor asked.

"Well, do you think Mother is in her right mind?"

Dr. Bishop thought for a moment, then responded: "Well, yes, in a certain sense. She is oriented to time and place, and she knows both her condition and the consequences of acting or not acting. But," he continued, "I wonder, personally, whether any person is in her right mind who refuses such a simple procedure when it will obviously save her life."

"I agree, Doctor, and I am willing to take the risk of getting the court involved. I will call my stateside lawyer tomorrow to see if he can convince the probate judge to appoint me as her guardian."

ADVANCE DIRECTIVES

"George," Jennifer spoke softly as she switched off the television special, "if anything like that ever happened to me, I wouldn't want to be hooked up to a bunch of machines." She looked at her husband of twenty years. "You wouldn't let them do that to me, would you?"

"No, honey," George replied, "if that's the way you feel."

"But, promise me," she insisted.

"Okay," he said, "but isn't it sometimes more complicated? For instance, suppose you get pneumonia and you need help breathing, and the doctor wants to use a respirator for a few days to give the drugs a chance to work? Or suppose you have an allergic reaction or something?"

"Well," Jennifer responded, "in that case I suppose it would be okay; but I wouldn't want it to go on forever, or to have to be dependent on it to breathe. What I mean is, if I had an accident or a stroke or something like that, if I didn't know what was happening or didn't have any hope of recovering, I wouldn't want to be kept alive by artificial means. I mean, once they hook you up, it can last a long time . . . and what's the use? I would just be a burden, and you couldn't really call that existence living."

Unfortunately, most people never have such a frank discussion of these issues, a discussion which makes it much easier for close relatives or friends to make a "substituted judgment" decision for them if necessary.

In most circumstances, however, it is even better to have a written statement expressing your personal desires, which can guide a substitute decision-maker. There are two forms of written advance directives. When Jennifer checked with her pastor, she was pleased to discover this form, which was available through the church:

THE CHRISTIAN'S LIVING WILL
To My Family, Physician, Clergy, Attorney, or Medical Facility:

First: I, _____, as a Christian, believe that "whether we live or die, we belong to the Lord" (Romans 14:8). If death is certain, so is the faithfulness of God in death as in life. With this high hope to sustain me, I wish to be as responsible in dying as in living.

Second: To this end, I implore all those responsible for my care and knowledgeable of my condition to be completely honest with me in the event of a terminal illness, that I may make my own decisions and preparations as much as possible.

Third: If there is no reasonable expectation of my recovery and I am no longer able to share decisions concerning my future, I ask that I be allowed to die and not be kept alive indefinitely by artificial means or heroic measures. I ask that drugs be administered to me as needed to relieve terminal suffering even if this may hasten the moment of my death. I am not asking that my life be directly taken, but that my dying be not unreasonably prolonged if my condition is hopeless, my deterioration irreversible, and the maintenance of my life an overwhelming responsibility for my family or an unfair monopoly of medical resources.

Fourth: This request is made thoughtfully while I am in good health and spirits. Even if this document be not binding legally, I beg those who care for me to honor its intent, which is in part to relieve them of some of the burden of this decision. In this way, I take responsibility for my own death and gladly give my life back to God.

(Copyrighted 1975 by New Samaritan Communications Corporation)

A "Living Will" is essentially an expression of the signer's philosophy. Unless amended, it does not give specific instructions. And, in its standard form, it actually applies in only a very narrow set of circumstances; specifically, to patients who are imminently dying. Many permanently incompetent patients, however, are not terminally ill—for example, patients with Alzhiemer's disease may live for many years. Even though it is not legally binding in some states, a living will could be taken as an expression of a patient's desire that not all therapies be continued as long as possible. In Jennifer's case, her physician filed the living will in his office chart and assured her that he understood her wishes.

Power of Attorney

A *Power of Attorney* is a legal document that a person (called the principal) signs to assign specific authority to another person (called his agent) to do a specific task (e.g., sell a house, sign checks, etc.). The power automatically terminates if the principal becomes incompetent. A *Durable Power of Attorney* is a similar document, but its authority continues even if the principal becomes incompetent.

A *Durable Power of Attorney for Health Care* (DPA/HC) is a new legal document being introduced in several states. It is designed specifically to name an agent to act on behalf of the principal in making health care decisions. It takes effect only when the principal becomes incompetent. Some DPA/HCs only name the agent, and others specify what types of treatments the principal would like given or omitted in what circumstances. It is obviously a more flexible document than the Living Will and can be more useful to a physician seeking help with a decision for an incompetent person. It is a lot easier explaining treatment options to a live person (the agent) and asking for a decision than it is reading a piece of paper that may or may not apply in the present situation.

For instance, when Jennifer signed her Living Will, she did not realize that there is a legal and ethical controversy (see the chapters on euthanasia and nutrition) regarding whether the provision of food and water through a tube is sustaining life by "artificial means," the term used in her document. If the situation occurred where her life depended on tube feeding, but she was not terminally ill, would she want to be kept alive by tube feeding? There is more flexibility if she has verbally expressed her convictions to a person than if she tries to antici-pate all possibilities in writing, including changing medical and legal definitions and practice. The advantage of the Living Will, however, is that it states her wishes in a formal, written form. These two types of advance directives can be effectively combined. For example, the Living Will can outline a person's general wishes regarding end-of-life treatment. In the Living Will, the person can also specify a person or persons who can act as a durable power of attorney and can interpret the Liv-ing Will to help make technical, moment-to-moment medical decisions.

Summary of Concepts

- Treatment decisions require the valid consent of a com-petent patient or surrogate.
- It is wise to anticipate possible incompetence and to designate a surrogate in that event.
- It is helpful to provide guidance to that substitute so the decisions made will be most consistent with your wishes.
- This guidance can be verbal, but written guidance is better, and designating a person to interpret the writ-ten guidance is best.

A BIBLICAL PERSPECTIVE

As with many subjects in medical ethics, the Bible does not specifically address the question of consent and competence. There are, however, some principles that provide guidance:

- God is sovereign. He has ultimate authority over life and death. In life or in death, we are the Lord's (Romans 9:19-24, 14:8).
- At the same time, He has given us free will, and He allows us to make decisions that are not His desire (Matthew 7:13-14).
- We are stewards of our own bodies and lives, and we're responsible to use them for His honor and glory while we have life (1 Corinthians 6:20).
- We are to take care of ourselves and our loved ones, whether it be "honoring our father and mother" (Deuteronomy 5:16) or providing for the needs of relatives (1 Timothy 5:8).
- We are to live healthful lifestyles and to seek medical care when needed.
- We are also stewards of our health-care resources and are to use them wisely.

When confronted with life-and-death decisions, we are to remember that human life is precious; it is a gift from God. Whether we are happy with our lot or not, we also know that there may be value in suffering. Finally, by faith, we know human life is not the greatest good to be clutched after at all costs—for in the end, with the Apostle Paul, we would prefer "to be away from the body and at home with the Lord" (2 Corinthians 5:8).

As Christians, we have the advantage of the Holy Spirit who is our comforter and help as we wrestle with life's more difficult decisions. His guiding presence and comfort assures us that whatever we decide, we decide under God's wings.

FOR DISCUSSION

Opening: Give everyone a chance to tell which (if any) of the following situations they have ever experienced:

___ Deciding the treatment or non-treatment of an unconscious relative.

___ Making medical decisions for a minor.

___ Deciding how much a relative should be told about his or her condition.

___ Feeling that your doctor and/or family is not giving you all the facts about your condition and options.

___ Facing resistance from your doctor and/or family about a decision you've made regarding your own medical treatment.

___ Disagreeing with a patient/relative/friend about his or her treatment decision.

___ Making your own Living Will.

___ Having to follow someone else's Living Will.

___ Being a legal guardian or durable power of attorney.

1. Recall the difficult treatment decision faced by John's parents (pages 82-83). Their options are:

   • Try surgery, which might cause further brain damage but might allow John to live for years in his persistent vegetative state.
   • Repeatedly administer antibiotics until they lose effectiveness, in which case he would probably die within a few weeks.
   • Stop antibiotics now, knowing he would die from the infection within several days.

   a. What would you do, and why?
   b. What principles of ethics apply here? (See the list on page 96.)
   c. What biblical principles apply?

d. Would you involve anyone else in deciding? If so, who?

2. The judge in Nelly's case (pages 88-89) has temporarily postponed a decision on Jim's petition. The judge has asked everyone involved to meet and come to a decision. Present are Nelly, Robert (representing the local children), Jim (who has flown home for the meeting), Dr. Bishop, a social worker who knows Nelly well, and the chaplain of the nursing home where Nelly lives. For a group discussion, have different individuals role-play this meeting.

3. Suppose the court has actually intervened in Nelly's case, and you have been appointed her temporary legal guardian. How will you decide whether or not to proceed with the amputation? Do you think she has a right to refuse, knowing it will probably bring about her death?

4. You have had a stroke, and the prognosis is guardedly optimistic that you will recover, though you may never walk again. Because at present you cannot swallow, your spouse is faced with the decision of whether you should be kept alive by a feeding tube or perhaps intravenous feedings. If you could speak, what would you say?

5. Why do you think the Living Will is growing in popularity?

___ It protects from unlimited costs.
___ It expresses personal desires and philosophy.
___ It lets a person die with dignity.
___ It helps the family know what the person wants, so they won't have guilt feelings about "not having done everything possible."
___ It takes a little power away from the money-hungry doctors.
___ Other (name it).

6. What do you think of a Living Will? Do you have one, or do you plan to complete one in the future?

NOTES:
1. Jay Katz, *The Silent World of Doctor and Patient* (New York: The Free Press, 1984).
2. James F. Childress and Mark Siegler, "Metaphors and Models of Doctor-Patient Relationships: Their Implications for Autonomy," *Theoretical Medicine,* February 1984, 5:17-30.
3. Judith Areen, "The Legal Status of Consent Obtained from Families of Adult Patients to Withhold or Withdraw Treatment," *Journal of the American Medical Association,* 1987, 258:229-235.
4. Lawrence J. Schneiderman and John D. Arras, "Counseling Patients to Counsel Physicians on Future Care in the Event of Patient Incompetence," *Annals of Internal Medicine,* May 1985, 102:693-698.

Chapter Six

The Plague

"I can't believe you're telling me this," Bill said. "How could I have AIDS?"

"Bill, I wish there were an easier answer to your symptoms," Dr. Kilmer continued, trying to help his personal friend adjust to this devastating news. At first he himself hadn't believed the results. "But we ran it three times," he continued, "and all three tests were positive for HIV, the AIDS virus."

"But I'm not a homosexual! You know that. You know me as well as anybody. I've never had sex with anyone but my wife!" His thoughts turned to Nancy. "Oh, please," he said, his head in his hands. "That means Nancy. . . ."

"I'm sorry, Bill," Dr. Kilmer continued softly. "She'll need to be tested, too. But there's a good chance she may have a negative test."

"And the baby?" Bill asked. They were expecting in three months.

"That depends," the doctor spoke quietly. "If Nancy is negative, the baby is safe. If not, there's a fifty-fifty chance." Dr. Kilmer paused. "I've combed your medical records, and my conclusion is that it must have been that blood transfusion you had. That's important to know, but right now it's not the most important thing. We've got to deal with the fact of this illness. We've got to do more tests and find out how your body is reacting to the virus. And Nancy will have to come in, too. The other kids should be safe."

"But, Frank," Bill pleaded, searching his friend's face for some hope, "there must be some mistake. I can't have AIDS." But looking into the doctor's eyes, he knew it was true, and the revelation began to sink in.

At the time of this diagnosis, Bill Stamfield was a thirty-four-year-old, middle-level executive—a likeable, outgoing young man. He had an undergraduate degree in Japanese from the University of California (San Francisco) and an MBA from the University of Chicago. He had been doing well in business, particularly in promoting his company's products in the Pacific Rim.

Bill Stamfield's family included three children, and another child was on the way. He had always enjoyed excellent health. His only medical problem had been a ruptured spleen from a car accident in 1984 when he had been in San Francisco on company business. He then underwent surgery and was given two units of blood.

At that time, in San Francisco, the risk of getting the AIDS virus from a blood transfusion was one in four hundred. There was no way to test for the virus (since 1985 there has been a test for the antibody to the virus, and blood supplies for transfusions are almost completely free of the virus now because of this test).

Bill's job performance also had been excellent. His evaluations were superb. His boss had been considering him for a promotion, but one day he noticed Bill looking pale and haggard. He had obviously lost weight. Over the next several months, Bill began to use sick leave. His direct supervisor began to notice that his work output was deteriorating. The supervisor confronted Bill about the use of alcohol or drugs, but Bill vehemently denied abusing these substances.

Bill had already been to his personal doctor, but he had not told his company the results of his HIV antibody test. His supervisors thought his problem was due to stress from frequent travel.

One day Bill became sick at work, fainted, and the company physician came to examine him. Bill showed evidence of weight loss and had swollen lymph glands in several areas, including his neck and under his arms. The company physician became concerned about some type of malignancy, like lymphoma, or even AIDS, and suggested appropriate tests be done.

Bill then admitted to the company physician and his supervisor that his private physician had been treating him for AIDS. Bill was placed in a less stressful job but was allowed to continue working for the company.

In the meantime, his supervisor struggled with several issues. Should he ask Bill to tell his fellow employees? Does Bill present any risk of infection to them?

Bill became increasingly ill over the next eight months, despite the use of the antiviral drug called Azidothymidine (AZT). During this period, his wife tested positive for HIV as well. Their son was born, and he also tested positive for HIV.

As his disease progressed, Bill developed both pneumocystis carinii, a severe lung infection, and Kaposi's sarcoma, a cancer which can spread throughout the body of an AIDS patient. These and other AIDS-related diseases are called "opportunistic," because they take the opportunity to overwhelm a depressed immune system. By contrast, the immune system of a normally healthy human is able to handle these infections and cancers quite easily. This is why the AIDS-related infections are uncommon among patients without AIDS. Also, the presence of these rare infections make AIDS relatively easy to diagnose.

Nine months after receiving the AIDS diagnosis, Bill was hospitalized with another severe bout of pneumocystis pneumonia and placed on an artificial breathing machine. Despite treatment, Bill's condition worsened. At one point he motioned to the doctors that things were on the "up and up," but he never was taken off the ventilator.

One week later, Bill Stamfield died. His supervisor was deeply grieved, and his company was saddened by his death.

During his illness, his company never thought about Bill's hospitalization costs as a factor in his medical decision-making. Later, however, the supervisor learned that Bill's total hospital debt was $152 thousand, and including the outpatient treatment and AZT, his health care costs ran over $200 thousand.

In addition, Bill's wife and their newborn son, possibly developing AIDS as well, were requiring medical treatment for HIV. The present impact and future implications of this single illness on the company's insurance plan were significant. The supervisor discussed the situation with the chief executive officer of the company.

"Mr. Schmidt, I just don't know how we should handle these cases in the future. Should we—can we legally—test all future employees for HIV to avoid another episode like this? I know this was a special case, and Bill's auto accident might even be viewed as work-related, but blood transfusions are safer now . . . and I don't know how we could be blamed for that, anyway." He stopped for a moment, remembering the agony his employee had endured. "And what about his family? What are we going to do about Mrs. Stamfield and her newborn son in terms of paying for their medical treatment?"

Mr. Schmidt was well-known for his decisive mind and quick answers. But this time he just sat back in his swivel chair and played with his letter opener. "I don't know," he said quietly. "I don't know." After a long pause, Mr. Schmidt asked, "How much money will it cost to pay for AZT for Bill's wife and son?" The supervisor shrugged his shoulders. "I'm not sure. I hear it's about $6 thousand a year just for the pills alone."

Mr. Schmidt made a decision. "Try to get them off our policy under the pre-existing disease clause," he ordered.

AIDS—A WORLDWIDE EPIDEMIC

AIDS (Acquired Immunodeficiency Syndrome) is a "new" disease (first described in 1981) that results from infection with the human immunodeficiency virus (HIV). The HIV is spread through sexual intercourse and exchange of infected body fluids, particularly blood.[1] Once infection occurs, it may be a long time before the patient actually gets AIDS. A fatal illness, AIDS is characterized by depressed immunity, a bewildering array of infections and cancers and, in many cases, *dementia*.[2]

As of 1990, some ninety thousand cases of AIDS were reported in the United States, and by 1991 the total will be 150 thousand. In San Francisco the number of deaths from AIDS by the end of the 1990s will exceed that city's death toll from all the wars of the twentieth century. As Bill discovered, even getting a blood transfusion in San Francisco before 1985 was a high risk; estimates are that as many as half of all homosexual men in San Francisco have the virus.

As many as one and a half million Americans are infected with the HIV. AIDS has been reported in all age groups, including children and the elderly. Over seventy percent of the cases have occurred in homosexual or bisexual men; twenty percent in intravenous drug abusers; two percent in people who received contaminated blood; one percent in people with *hemophilia*; and the remainder in heterosexuals or persons who died before complete histories could be obtained.[3] AIDS is more than a syndrome. It is a plague. Webster's dictionary defines plague as "Any epidemic disease that is deadly."

AIDS is already a severe problem in central Africa, where heterosexual and intrauterine (inside the womb) transmission of the disease is common. About one in ten persons are infected (extreme poverty makes it difficult to estimate the true incidence). Dr. Jonathan Mann, World Health Organization (WHO) Coordinator for AIDS, is concerned that the severity of the epidemic in the two-thirds world could force the WHO to abandon much of its critical work on measles, malnutrition, and childhood diarrhea.[4]

By the year 2000, every second adult in Uganda will be HIV-positive. In Rwanda, children account for twenty percent of AIDS cases, and six thousand AIDS babies are expected to be born this year in Zambia. Of eight hundred prostitutes tested in Nairobi, nine out of ten were HIV-positive, and each claimed an average of one thousand customers per year. WHO speculates that as many as fifty to one hundred million people worldwide will be HIV-infected by 1991, with more than three million reported AIDS cases.

There will be a geographic spread of the HIV infection, and even if a vaccine becomes available in the West (which researchers say is highly unlikely), it will take decades before it becomes available to most of the world's population.

As if all this weren't bad enough news, some AIDS cases found in Africa have been identified as being caused by another AIDS virus: HIV-2. This virus is related to but genetically different from HIV-1. The researchers who reported on its discovery in the *New England Journal of Medicine* fear that HIV-2 will eventually spread into the west.

AIDS TESTING

Methods

The ELISA test for AIDS involves the use of an enzyme to test for the body's antibody to the human immunodeficiency virus. The test does not reveal the virus itself, but the body's reaction to it. The body can take some time to react to the virus—weeks, months, even years—so the test is negative at first, even if a patient is infected with the virus. If the ELISA is positive, the Western Blot test is used to confirm the ELISA.

The Western Blot finds antibodies that are more specific for the HIV than the ELISA test, so it is less likely to give a false positive result. The cost of testing varies, but it is usually less than fifteen dollars.

Who Should Be Tested?
The following people are at risk:

- People with symptoms suggesting AIDS-Related Complex (ARC) or AIDS.
- Any man who has had intercourse with another man since 1977.
- People who use intravenous drugs and share needles.
- People who use non-intravenous drugs but have promiscuous sex, which is often associated with the use of these drugs.
- People from Haiti or Central Africa.
- Prostitutes and their sexual partners.
- People planning to get married or thinking about having a child if they have not been in a monogamous relationship for seven or more years.
- Missionaries who have worked in the two-thirds world and may have been exposed to blood or blood products or contaminated syringes.

THE TRANSMISSION OF AIDS

Sixteen-year-old Shawna has been thinking about having sex with seventeen-year-old Andy. It would be her first sexual experience. But what she doesn't know is that Andy has had sexual intercourse with Susan, who has previously had sex with Brian. Susan didn't know that Brian had been an intravenous drug abuser in the past and that he carries the AIDS virus.

Unknown to her, if Shawna goes ahead and sleeps with Andy, she will become connected, by a web of sexual contacts, to someone who has the virus. Whether or not she will get the virus depends on how many in the group actually became infected by the virus and whether she herself contracts the HIV from her involvement with Andy.

AIDS is harder to get than most sexually transmitted diseases. But careful studies have proven that the virus, like gonorrhea and other sexually transmitted diseases, can and does spread through the web of sexual contacts. Thus, on her very first sexual contact, Shawna would have a small risk of contracting AIDS.

The human immunodeficiency virus can infect and damage many types of cells, especially white blood cells of the immune system. HIV can also attack many other tissues, including the vagina, cervix, male and female urethra, rectum, and brain. In the cells of these tissues, HIV is incorporated directly into the DNA, which stores the genetic code.

Effective transmission of the virus may require the transfer of significant quantities of white blood cells infected with HIV and free viral particles. Semen, vaginal fluid, and blood of infected persons can contain large numbers of both infected white cells and viral particles. Small scrapes and cuts that occur during sex may allow the exchange of both infected secretions and blood. Perhaps this explains why the AIDS virus, although it is present in most body fluids including saliva, is transmitted *most effectively* during rectal or vaginal intercourse and through blood transfusions or contaminated needles and syringes.

Since mother and child are in intimate contact, another and increasingly common mode of transmission is from infected mothers to infants in the womb, during birth, and through breast-feeding.

When AIDS is spread through sex, it first spreads most quickly among the most promiscuous members of the population, and then it moves through the rest of the population more slowly. In Africa, heterosexuals are more promiscuous than homosexuals, so AIDS in Africa is a heterosexual disease. In Africa, the numbers of male and female AIDS cases are about equal.

In America, the disease initially spread through the homosexual population. AIDS is now slowly spreading through the heterosexual population in America, just like it has always spread in Africa. Women are the new risk group. The number of reported female AIDS cases is increasing in our country, predominantly through shared contaminated needles or sexual intercourse with bisexual male partners. The proportion of female AIDS victims who reported transmission through heterosexual contact has more than doubled since 1982—from twelve percent of all cases in women to twenty-six percent of cases in women. The virus is transmitted from women to men and vice versa during vaginal intercourse. Penile penetration is not required. In fact, there is a case in which lesbian sex has been implicated in the transmission of the virus.

Besides transmission through sexual activity, AIDS can also be transmitted through nonsexual means, usually involving a contaminated blood transfusion or a doctor or nurse sticking themselves with a needle used on an HIV-positive patient.

A second-year resident working on a bone marrow transplantation unit in 1983 was performing a lab test on his patient. The tube containing the blood shattered and some blood and glass penetrated the doctor's finger. Three weeks later, the doctor became acutely ill with a rash, cough, and sore throat. The illness resolved, and the resident went on to become a cardiologist. He married, and the couple had a child. But in 1986 he began losing weight, felt tired, and had many other symptoms. He was then tested for AIDS. The test was positive. A test of the stored blood from the now-deceased bone marrow transplant patient was also positive.[5]

While doctors can rarely "get AIDS" at work, the overwhelming evidence is that household contacts, school contacts, and other casual human contacts *do not* transmit the virus. Like syphilis, the virus requires intimate, person-to-person contact for transmission. Coughs, sneezes, kisses, toothbrushes, towels, toilet seats, utensils, air, and food can't transmit the disease.

WHAT AIDS PATIENTS EXPERIENCE

AIDS patients develop parasitic pneumonias, fungal meningitis, widespread tuberculosis, disseminated herpes, and unusual cancers like Kaposi's sarcoma. Wasting (in Africa, AIDS is called "slim disease") and death occur within several years in most cases. ARC seems in many patients to precede or supersede the full-blown syndrome of AIDS. Estimates of the number of ARC patients vary, but as many as 210 thousand persons in the United States and as many as five million worldwide are currently thought to have ARC. ARC can also be rapidly fatal. The fate of patients who are HIV-positive but have no signs of disease is still uncertain, but most, if not all, will eventually develop ARC or AIDS and die.

While many of the individual diseases associated with AIDS can be treated, they often occur in combination, and there is no effective cure for the underlying disease itself. Bill, for example, had two different kinds of pneumonia and three different kinds of germs causing diarrhea. When his doctors tried to treat several of these at once, he developed side effects to the medicines they were giving him. The only medicine that really helped him was AZT.

Now available on the market, AZT has proven to be beneficial in prolonging life. But the best this drug can do is turn a rapidly fatal disease into a more chronic, but still fatal, disease. Unfortunately, AZT can't reverse the underlying immune system destruction caused by the virus. AZT has also shown promise in postponing the development of full-blown AIDS in patients with ARC or patients who are still early in their course of HIV-infection. Many other drugs designed to boost the immune system are currently in the early testing phase.

While somewhat promising, and certainly better than nothing, AZT is toxic and expensive. Ten to twenty percent of those treated with AZT develop anemia, and some require ongoing transfusions. AZT must be taken for the rest of the patient's life.

THE COST OF AIDS

Despite America's wealth, treatment for AIDS is more expensive than we can imagine. In 1985 the number of hospitalized AIDS patients was 5,395, the average length of stay was nineteen days, and the total cost was $380 million. By 1991, the care of AIDS patients will cost nearly $12 billion yearly.[6] Public teaching hospitals—which, like hospitals in the two-thirds world, are already overburdened—will be most adversely affected.

AIDS AS A PLAGUE: AN ANALYSIS

The AIDS plague has similarities to other scourges. Persons with AIDS are as severely stigmatized as lepers, but their illness often evokes less compassion because the transmission characteristics of AIDS are like those of syphilis. AIDS has the natural history of tuberculosis, with a long incubation period and a relatively slow, wasting course. AIDS also has the prognosis of untreated bubonic plague—certain death.

In times of plague, people learn firsthand about the scale of an epidemic's tragedy and horror. Our encounters with AIDS force us to make difficult choices. They are choices we each will have to make, because AIDS is no longer confined to a certain geographic area; AIDS is an epidemic. We are faced with choices as old as time itself: to desert, to persecute, or to show compassion.

Desertion

In plague times of the Middle Ages, many Christians, including physicians and clergy, deserted the cities and their poor and dying inhabitants. During the plague of 1665, most of

London's wealthy citizens and nearly all of the physicians fled. Almost seventy thousand of the four-hundred thousand citizens died. Due to the mass exodus of physicians, records indicate there were only thirteen doctors to care for the more than two-hundred thousand Londoners who remained in the city.[7]

Desertion has also characterized some modern physicians' and dentists' responses to HIV-infected patients. A prominent heart surgeon has stated publicly that he will refuse to operate on HIV-infected individuals.[8] Some physicians and dentists quietly "refer" them. Many families and some communities have also been reluctant to care for HIV-infected persons. AIDS is increasingly becoming a disease of the urban poor and minorities. The bulk of actual health care for AIDS victims falls upon interns and residents in overloaded public hospitals.

Desertion in medieval plague times, combined with the severity of the plagues, often resulted in near-total collapse of society. Disorder, violence, and malnutrition were common, and these conditions made the population more susceptible to the plague. The consequences of deserting AIDS patients are analogous. In Central Africa, AIDS seems destined to shatter societies already compromised by malnutrition, poverty, and other diseases. In America, while the situation is far less serious, our spiritual, physical, and financial desertion of AIDS patients may also aggravate the plague.

Persecution

In the book entitled *The City of God,* Saint Augustine points to the tendency during plague time to assign blame and persecute the scapegoats. Raymond Crawfurd, in *Plague and Pestilence in Literature and Art,* provides a frightening picture of the process:

> Amid all the panic of the Black Death, persecution [of certain minorities] broke out. . . . Some victim was needed to appease the maddened populace . . . they were

accused of poisoning the wells, and even of infecting the air. Circumstantial accounts were circulated throughout Europe of secret operations . . . and the concoction of poisons from spiders, owls, and other supposed venomous animals was described.[9]

In Milan, Italy, in 1630, two men—a barber-surgeon and the commissioner of health—were accused of spreading the plague by means of deadly ointments. The senate decreed that their flesh should be torn with red-hot pincers, their right hands cut off, their bones broken, and that they should be put on the wheel for six hours, then burned at the stake.

While such actions are unthinkable today, there are still vestiges of the persecution model in effect. We no longer cut off arms and legs—just employment and benefits! For instance, some patients have been summarily fired from their jobs when it was learned that they were HIV-positive. Haitians were accused of importing the epidemic to the United States, but recent studies indicate the opposite is true! School children who are HIV-positive have been forced to leave their schools, and in several cases, forced to leave town. One family's home was destroyed by arson.

Jeff wondered why AIDS patients couldn't just be isolated from the rest of the population. "I would make sure every American was tested, and I would put all the positives in isolation," he insisted.

"But AIDS isn't spread through coughing," Gordon protested. "Isolation may work for a disease which can be easily spread and lasts only a short time. But I don't think it would be right to keep people in isolation for the rest of their lives. Some HIV-positive persons might live for many years before they develop AIDS."

"Then why not tattoo the positives?" Jeff responded.

Gordon shook his head. "You don't understand. This disease is spread in bedrooms through sex or on the street through the use of illegal drugs. Millions of Americans will eventually have the virus. It is a slow virus. We just can't isolate everybody. Let me put it this way, if you can't understand it any other way. It will cost billions of dollars to isolate and police all of these people. I am not willing to pay the price of this isolation, either in human terms or in actual dollars."

Jeff shrugged his shoulders. "I still think we should put these people away."

During the Black Plague, the maddened populace sealed up their own springs and wells and had to rely on rain and river water. They also killed their own physicians. The consequences of modern persecution of persons who are HIV-positive are analogous. Adequate treatment of the disease, and the prevention of further spread, depends on the cooperation of those who are HIV-positive or at risk.

Dr. Hallworth is a public health official who has learned that an HIV-positive individual is continuing to have unprotected sexual intercourse with multiple individuals. Dr. Hallworth has the difficult task of balancing the rights of HIV-infected versus HIV-uninfected individuals. As a public health official, however, his goal is clear. He is to protect the general health of the public, even if that means taking some sort of restraining action against this particular HIV-infected person. In this case he successfully pursues legal action to bring the HIV-positive person into the health-care setting for counseling and further observation.

The choices to desert and persecute have similar consequences. The poor and the plague-prone become disenfranchised. The population becomes fragmented and demoralized. The plague spreads.

Compassion

Throughout history, there were notable Christians who were exceptions to desertion and persecution. Pope Clement VI extended his personal protection to persecuted minorities at Avignon. William Boghurst remained to care for patients during a severe plague in England. He deplored the desertion by those who could help attend the plague victims, and he wrote that everyone who is a professional must take the benefits and responsibilities together. Ministers must preach, captains must fight, physicians must attend to the sick.

During the 1793 epidemic of yellow fever in Philadelphia, most of the physicians fled. But Benjamin Rush, a Christian doctor, remained. The reason he gave was that he had a duty to care for his patients even at the jeopardy of his own life.

In the few plagues in which compassion was extended to those in trouble, the societies experienced less deterioration than during times of desertion or persecution. The people did not lose confidence in the professions and institutions, including the church. The terror was overcome, and eventually the plague passed or diminished in scope.

If persons with AIDS are treated with compassion, their suffering will be eased, societal disruption will be lessened, and a frightened culture will see an example of Christian love. In a society where many may turn away from AIDS patients in the next few years, the AIDS plague presents a special opportunity to the church to minister in the name of the One who touched the lepers and ministered to the disenfranchised of His own day, Jesus of Nazareth.

CLINICAL NOTES OF A FORMER PHARISEE

Understanding the need for compassion toward those with AIDS ultimately requires knowing someone who has the disease. Dr. Schiedermayer learned much from caring for his first patient with AIDS, a man named James. This is Dr. Schiedermayer's story:

> At first I tried to dismiss James' disease because he acquired HIV infection from promiscuous homosexual activity. But as I saw what the virus did to him clinically—destroying his immune system, causing him to lose a third of his body weight, infiltrating his

brain—I realized that AIDS is like other diseases, other plagues. When this plague passes, another will come, with different initials and perhaps a different mode of transmission. As long as there are people, there will be diseases and plagues.

AIDS can bring out the Pharisee in us. One of my first thoughts, when I began taking care of James, was to thank God that I was not like him. And then I remembered the moral Jesus added at the end of the parable of the Pharisee and the publican: "Everyone who exalts himself will be humbled, and he who humbles himself will be exalted" (Luke 18:14).

The Bible does not condone homosexual practices; they are considered, like many of the things we do, sinful. But in treating AIDS patients we may begin despising them, thinking ourselves to be righteous in comparison to them. I began my treatment of James with the attitude of a Pharisee, thanking God that I was "not like other men." I tried to see his disease as somehow different from other diseases, and I did not consider the possibility that this stigmatized man had repented or wished to repent. In my heart, I approved of his suffering and inevitable death.

I count my attitude as sin equal to his—no, as greater sin, according to Jesus, if the patient repents. I have been able to change my mind about AIDS and persons with HIV infection. I seek to be like Him who touched lepers and prostitutes, who took the blame, who bears the stigma. Yet I still feel the struggle of the plague doctor within me, the doctor whose stark choices are desertion, persecution, or compassion.[10]

FOR DISCUSSION

Opening: In the next few years, everyone will know someone who has AIDS or has already died from the disease. Have group members describe any experiences they have had with this situation.

1. Your six-year-old daughter comes home from school announcing that a new boy in her first-grade class has AIDS. He has just moved to town with his two sisters and brother from California, to live with their uncle, John Stamfield, and his family in your small town in New Hampshire. You had heard through the grapevine that both parents of these children had died from AIDS, and now those rumors seem more credible. What will you do?
   a. Pull your daughter out of that school.
   b. Call the principal and demand that the boy be pulled out of school.
   c. Nothing.
   d. Call or send a note to the Stamfield family, expressing your deep sympathy and offering any support.
   e. Instruct your daughter about the risks of the disease.
   f. Other (name it).

2. Your church board has asked for input from church members about the possible development of a ministry to AIDS patients in the community. Which of these questions do you think ought to be discussed?
   a. Is there really a need?
   b. How are such ministries organized elsewhere?
   c. What positive or negative impact has this outreach had elsewhere?
   d. What resources are required: financial, personnel, etc.?
   e. What is an appropriate Christian response to these persons?
   f. How might these persons respond to religious groups getting involved?
   g. Other (explain).

3. Proposals for AIDS prevention have caused conflict between

the scientific community and the religious community. Science would prevent transmission primarily by condom and spermicide use; the religious community would prevent transmission primarily by premarital chastity and marital monogamy.

    a. Is there any common ground? How do you think the spread of the epidemic can best be curbed?

    b. Read Numbers 16:46-48. Can Christians act as a living barrier to the spread of the AIDS virus?

4. Considering the projected costs ($12 billion annually) by 1991, and the likelihood that these costs will be paid by the taxpayers:

    a. Do you think AIDS patients should be treated as aggressively as leukemia patients?

    b. How would you begin to establish limits?

    c. What if the patient wanted more aggressive treatment than society was willing to provide?

5. Read about some of the plagues recorded for us in the Bible (Exodus 32:35; Numbers 11:33, 14:37, 16:41-50; Joshua 22:17; 1 Samuel 5:8-12; 2 Samuel 24:10-25; Revelation 11:6, 15:1-8, 16:1-21, 22:18-19).

    Note that many seem to have been sent as a judgment. Is the plague of AIDS a judgment? Would God send plagues among the innocent as well as the guilty?

NOTES:
1. Thomas A. Peterman and James W. Curran, "Sexual Transmission of Human Immunodeficiency Virus," *Journal of the American Medical Association,* October 24-31, 1986, 256:2222-2226.
2. David D. Ho, Roger J. Pomerantz, and Joan C. Kaplan, "Pathogenesis of Infection with Human Immunodeficiency Virus," *New England Journal of Medicine,* July 30, 1987, 317:278-286.
3. Centers for Disease Control, "Human Immunodeficiency Virus Infection in the United States: A Review of Current Knowledge," *Mortality and Morbidity Weekly Reports* (supplement no. S-6, 1987), p. 36.
4. Jonathan M. Mann and James Chin, "AIDS: A Global Perspective," *New England Journal of Medicine,* August 4, 1988, 319:302-303.

5. Hacib Aoun, "When a House Officer Gets AIDS," *New England Journal of Medicine,* September 7, 1989, 321:693-696.
6. John K. Iglehart, "Financing the Struggle Against AIDS," *New England Journal of Medicine,* July 16, 1987, 317:180-184.
7. Warren G. Bell, *The Great Plague in London in 1665* (New York: Dodd Mead and Co., Inc., 1924).
8. "Heart Surgeon Won't Operate on Victims of AIDS," *New York Times,* March 12, 1987.
9. Raymond Crawfurd, *Plagues and Pestilence in Literature and Art* (Oxford, England: Clarendon Press, 1914).
10. David L. Schiedermayer, "Choices in Plague Time," *Christianity Today,* August 7, 1989, pp. 20-22.

Chapter Seven

The Final Years

"I'm sorry this is taking so long," the nurse apologized, "but we don't discharge patients very often. We're trying to round up the paperwork."

Just a month earlier, Jeff Davis's eighty-seven-year-old mother had entered Greenbriar Nursing Home. Until recently, Jeff's father had been caring for her at home. But she was becoming incontinent, and she often fell, sometimes hurting herself in the process. The most recent episode left her with two black eyes and a swollen face. Gradually, and very reluctantly, Jeff's father had concluded that he could no longer care for her at home.

Now, after these few weeks of nursing home placement, Grandpa Davis had reached another decision, one that he had previously resisted. He would accept his oldest son's offer to have them move in with his family. The nursing home care was very expensive, and Grandpa Davis didn't think his wife received enough attention. Unless he moved her quickly, judging by the first month's costs, their meager financial resources would be depleted very quickly.

As Jeff wheeled his mother to the car, he knew that the sacrifices it meant for his wife and children were certainly preferable to Grandma Davis spending her final days in a nursing home. She seemed happy to go with him, but then again, she seemed happy most of the time.

THE INCREASING NEED FOR LONG-TERM CARE (LTC)

Fortunately, not all elderly persons need nursing home care. The majority are able to remain independent or live with family members. Only six percent of the elderly in North America spend their last days in nursing homes. In 1989, 2.3 million people in the U.S. lived in nursing homes, a number that may double in the next thirty years.[1] Most of these patients are suffering from chronic diseases like arthritis, Parkinson's disease, and Alzheimer's disease. There are significant differences between acute and chronic illnesses.

COMPARISON OF CHRONIC AND ACUTE DISEASES

CHRONIC	ACUTE
•Chronic diseases are incurable and may result in significant disability.	•Acute diseases may be curable.
•The treatment goal is management, preserving function, forestalling complications.	•The treatment goal is restoration of health and function, reversing illness/injury.
•The illness is gradually perceived as a part of the person, to be negotiated with.	•The illness is seen as an external threat or force to be battled against.

Much "negotiating" with chronic illness takes place in the acute-care setting (physician's office, hospital, home). But many patients regress to the point of *debilitation* and require long-term institutional care.

Nursing homes have become increasingly sophisticated and increasingly incorporated into the medical care system. Previously they were considered more as alternative residences suited for those who required occasional nursing attention. But as medical advances have allowed us to prolong the lives of many patients who would have died in earlier generations, nursing homes have assumed the medical care of those with severe chronic illnesses. Furthermore, cost containment measures have encouraged the discharge of patients from hospitals "quicker and sicker." Many of these early discharges require short or long-term nursing home care. Nursing homes are now prepared to offer more than residential services. Many people in nursing homes are severely impaired in terms of ability to walk, to think, or to control their bowels and bladders.

Medical triumphs have reduced or eliminated many infectious diseases, postponed death from cancer, heart disease, and stroke, and in other ways made it possible for people to live longer. They are thus more likely to develop degenerative chronic diseases that result in disability.

Societal changes have given a major impetus to the nursing home industry. Earlier in the century, older people and those in need of care lived in the home. Society was primarily agrarian, with large homes and several children who usually lived in the same community after leaving home. Few wives worked outside the home, and unmarried adults often lived with the nuclear family.

In contrast, today's society is more urban or suburban and more mobile. Homes are smaller and families have fewer children. More wives work outside the home. Divorce is more frequent. Nonetheless, a large percentage of elderly patients (about sixty percent) still live with their children when they become ill or infirm. The amazing thing is that despite our mobile society, many of us in the "sandwich generation" care for both our children *and* our parents at home.

It is common to move grandmother or grandfather from another state to live with us. But after a series of strokes, or when Alzheimer's disease becomes severe, an aging parent may require more care than we can provide; then nursing home residence may be the only appropriate option.

An aging society, improved medical treatment for life-threatening diseases, and an inability to care for persons with degenerative conditions contribute to the need for more chronic-care beds, more sophisticated nursing home care, and the high cost of long-term care.

CHRONIC CARE RAISES ETHICAL QUESTIONS

Because chronic care has different goals and a different timetable than acute care, ethical issues in chronic care are different. Family members are often more involved with the management of chronic illness since many patients lack decision-making capacity. Thus, chronic illnesses may give us a different perspective of beneficence, confidentiality, and autonomy. Furthermore, institutional long-term care is very expensive; this raises questions about justice in distributing health-care resources.

In this chapter we will look at these ethical issues of chronic care: admission to a nursing home, payment for long-term care, the patient's rights, and treatment decisions.

Admission Decisions
I was always afraid it would end like this . . . even after everything I did for him. How can he do this to me? There must be another way. If only I could talk. . . .

"Now, Doctor," the son continued, as if his mother weren't even in the room, "we want nothing but the best for Mother. No matter how bad this gets, we always want her to be treated with respect and kindness." He glanced at his mother, lying in the hospital bed. There seemed to be a tear in her eye.

Nothing but the best? What about his place? But his wife would never hear of it. I fed him, changed his diapers a thousand times, but now a little inconvenience and they just want to put me away. She wanted to shout, but the words would not come out.

"Of course, we can't keep Mother at home in this condition, can we, Doctor? I mean, she needs much more time and special attention than Nancy could ever provide, considering her commitments to the church and charity groups. Besides, Nancy was never one for nursing. And with my work schedule, I certainly can't help much. So Cedar Ridge seems the best alternative, don't you think?"

Clinical and Social Factors

Usually, the decision to admit someone to a nursing home is based on the patient's loss of mobility, loss of bladder or bowel control, and/or mental confusion. The underlying disease may be arthritis, stroke, Alzheimer's disease, or some other degenerative condition.

Sometimes the reasons are social. For example, the person may not be able to provide self-care and has no family or friends who are willing or able to provide assistance in the home. Perhaps the person has outlived his or her spouse and children. Perhaps the home is not large enough to house the debilitated parent, or both caregivers in the home work. A final reason may be that the children do not feel any moral obligation to the parents because of their philosophical stance or because of divorce or other fractured family relationships.

But Whose Decision Is It?

When Aunt Rosalie fell and broke her hip, everyone (including Rosalie) agreed that it was no longer a good idea for her to live alone. She was eighty-two and infirm. A long-term care facility would be much safer for her.

Many decisions to admit patients to nursing homes arise from crises like a broken hip or a stroke. But often the loss of independent function is gradual, and the patient may deny such loss for a long time.

Dr. Garrett insisted that at seventy-two he could still do

surgery, until one day he left a surgical sponge inside a patient and the hospital decided it was time to force him to retire. A widower without any children, he continued living independently for the next five years, though visitors noticed the home was becoming unkempt. Dr. Garrett insisted on driving his car, despite his failing eyesight, until he was the cause of a near-fatal accident. Reluctantly, he accepted the advice of his doctor (and his lawyer) that he enter some type of long-term care facility.

The decision to move to a nursing home is often postponed as long as possible. Children, neighbors, friends, and physician may be ready for a person to be placed in a nursing home—but the patient may not yet be willing to go. This difference of opinion often generates friction, which may make the ultimate decision more difficult.

The patient's loss of decision-making capacity also makes nursing home placement a very difficult decision. *Dementia*, a process that affects about twenty-five percent of patients over age eighty-five, leads to irreversible loss of intellectual function. (See the appendix for a discussion of this common condition in the elderly.)

Benevolent Deceivers?

"Doctor," Tom said, "I feel I must make this decision for Mother for her own good. Will you help me by telling her that she needs to go into the hospital for some tests? She won't know it's actually a nursing home, and once we get her there, I hope she will agree to stay. Or if that won't work, maybe you could give her a sedative and we could move her while she is asleep."

Mrs. Henry was a widow. After her husband died, she rented out the upstairs bedrooms of her large comfortable home in a nice residential neighborhood. Her son Tom was attentive to her needs. He noticed that she was gradually becoming confused and was not as attentive regarding her appearance as she had been. Her tenants moved out one by one, confiding to the son that his mother was snooping into their things and was sounding bizarre in her conversation.

Whenever Tom suggested alternative living arrangements to his mother, she steadfastly maintained that she wanted to remain in her own home and take care of herself. Tom shopped for her, arranged for the delivery of one hot meal a day, and hired someone to clean her house. She remained quite healthy physically, but her mental function continued to deteriorate. She became paranoid, certain that the cleaning woman was stealing her belongings, fearful that the Meals-on-Wheels were poisoned, and convinced that Tom was trying to "put her away" so that he could take over her home.

Both Tom and his wife worked, and their home was not suitable for a live-in elderly person. Tom was convinced that his mother needed some sort of supervised living arrangement, and because of her mental deterioration, it seemed that a nursing home was necessary. But when Tom and his mother's physician had suggested this direction to Mrs. Henry, she adamantly refused to leave her home.

How were Tom and the doctor to proceed? Because of Mrs. Henry's refusal, should they just wait until she had a fall, got hurt, or developed some other physical disability? Or is it all right for Tom to take the decision out of his mother's hands? Does he need to petition the probate court for guardianship? Is it morally justifiable to lie to Mrs. Henry in order to pursue the greater good of looking out for her physical well-being?

Over the course of several years, Tom had been providing for his mother's needs, and in that process a child-parent role reversal had taken place. Some families make this adjustment easily and peacefully. Other families are plunged into power struggles that may uncover old, unresolved interpersonal conflicts. Fights may occur between parent and child. Siblings may quarrel over who gets to be in charge.

In Tom's case, it was his sister Julie who "threw in the monkey wrench," as he put it later. Just when he was determined to intervene, Julie (ten years younger, the baby of the family) came to town for her annual visit. Assuming they were allies in their mother's behalf, Tom told Julie he was having his lawyer draft the appropriate documents to ask the probate court to declare Mrs. Henry incompetent and make him her legal guardian.

The next thing Tom knew, Julie had told their mother all about it and together they had devised a counter-plan. Mother would sell the house and move to Cleveland with Julie. The proceeds of the house sale would establish a jointly owned trust fund to cover Mrs. Henry's living expenses. That arrangement lasted about two weeks until Mrs. Henry called the local police to report that Julie's husband was trying to steal her jewelry to pay the phone bill.

Payment for Long-Term Care

Mr. and Mrs. Kaul were in their early eighties, quite healthy, and very independent. They had both worked hard at low-paying jobs all their lives and had proudly accumulated $20 thousand in savings. Their combined social security and retirement checks were adequate for their needs, so they planned to leave the savings to their grandchildren. Then Mrs. Kaul had a stroke. Although alert, she was incontinent and totally paralyzed on her left side. She was not able to care for herself. In the hospital, Mr. Kaul tearfully sat in disbelief as the discharge planner explained to him his wife's need for a nursing home bed and the necessity to "spend down" their life savings before they could receive financial assistance. The discharge planner said that some people in this situation shield some of their savings by transferring it to a special trust fund. But the rules for this transfer were complicated, and Mr. Kaul wasn't sure it was ethical to avoid paying for his wife's care. He felt very confused as he tried to figure out what to do.

Most people are not able to afford the $2 thousand per month (average) cost of LTC for very long. Medicare pays only a small portion of such costs. Long-term care insurance is new and highly variable in quality; often coverage is incomplete.

Many who need protracted long-term care find it necessary to deplete their savings to the poverty level before the federally mandated, state-administered Medicaid program will step in and pay the bill. This process is painful and embarrassing for the patient, spouse, and family members.

Who Will Pay?

The major ethical question surrounding the financing of long-term care is: whose responsibility is it to pay? This question is not so much a question of medical ethics as it is a question of social justice. In the past, most families took care of their own infirm or ill elderly, and when they were unable to do so, the community and the church helped. Social and family changes and the current burgeoning population of infirm elderly have resulted in an increasing demand for long-term care. The present patchwork nonsystem of health care financing for long-term care now leaves the responsibility by default to the state, but only after the person in need meets poverty criteria.

What is the family's duty here? In Scripture, we read of Paul telling Timothy, "If anyone does not provide for his relatives, and especially for his immediate family, he has denied the faith and is worse than an unbeliever" (1 Timothy 5:8). Does he mean that adult children still have an obligation to provide financially for their parents? What is our response to the psalmist (or a parent) who cries, "Do not cast me away when I am old; do not forsake me when my strength is gone" (Psalm 71:9)? Does this imply financial obligation? If so, how do we set our priorities in regard to our children's needs (including the cost of education) versus the long-term care needs of our parents?

Some in our society believe the church still has a responsibility to provide facilities for those unable to care for themselves. The Apostle Paul instructs families to care for their own widows so they do not become a burden on the church, but then admonishes the church to care for those "widows who are really in need" (1 Timothy 5:16).

Other people believe that society has an obligation to

ensure that everyone is provided with a minimal standard of care at the end of their lives. Who decides what is a "minimal standard of care"? Or should it be more than minimal? The alternative to universal availability of long-term care is that the ability to pay will often determine the quality of care.

The long-term care facility may have obligations as well. Is it merely a business that must answer to its board or owners? Some facilities obligate themselves to hold current patients' beds if the patients are temporarily transferred to a hospital; but others fill the beds with paying patients as soon as possible. When two persons are in need of a bed but only one is available, some long-term care facilities consider payment method as a criterion for admission, but others give priority to the patient with the greatest need. The long-term care industry recognizes that the economic pressures of the marketplace mandate cost-consciousness. But our society, in the next decade or two, must address whether it is just to shift costs from medicaid to private insurers, or to other payment sources. Who pays when the patient cannot?

Beneficence Versus Justice

These ethical questions address the conflicts that arise between the principle of beneficence (doing what is best for the patient) and the principle of justice. Is long-term care a right or a privilege? How do individuals, families, and society distribute health-care dollars? If long-term care is a right, and if the government is partly responsible for payment, how can priorities be set to assure equitable distribution of limited resources? Who decides if a given medical community needs a new CT scanner or more nursing home beds?

The Patient's Rights

Mrs. James was a retired school teacher who had been widowed for many years. She enjoyed her retirement. She traveled quite a bit with old friends or "senior groups" and volunteered in several charity programs. She was close to her three married children and visited them often, even though they were geographically scattered.

Over the past five years, Mrs. James had become increasingly forgetful and unsteady on her feet. She had several falls, but no serious injuries. Her family convinced her to give up her apartment and live in an elderly housing complex which had an attached nursing home.

During her first month there, she had three falls; one resulted in a deep cut on her forehead, which required suturing. The nursing staff recommended that Mrs. James be moved to the intermediate care facility in the housing complex. The nurses there told Mrs. James she should call for assistance when she needed to get out of her chair. They are not sure if she merely forgot or was consciously refusing to call, but she fell again. Her physician agreed to the nursing supervisor's request for a soft-belt restraint to keep her in her chair and remind her to call for help. Mrs. James refused to have the restraint applied. The physician asked the family to become involved in convincing Mrs. James to accept the restraint for the sake of her own safety.

The limits on personal freedom required by long-term institutional care can be difficult for both patient and family to accept. Someone else determines the clothing worn, when and what to eat, what time (or even whether or not) to get up or go to bed, and how to spend leisure time. But the greatest conflict arises when the patient's freedom of movement is restricted.[2]

Mrs. James' case represents a conflict between the patient's right to self-determination (autonomy) and the health care provider's duty to do what is in the best interests of the patient (beneficence). What do you do when a patient's choices seem to put her safety, perhaps even her life, in jeopardy?

Other residents may be steady on their feet and in no danger of falling, but their forgetfulness may cause them to wander into rooms of other patients, to pick up others' food or possessions, and so on. Then their autonomy conflicts with the principle of justice. If some residents are granted their freedom of movement, then others may suffer in some regard.

Some patients may disrupt others by being argumentative, noisy, or inappropriately intimate. Should they be given medication to sedate them? Sometimes the sedation not only diminishes unwanted behavior, but also blunts their "joi de vivre."

Surveys of patients in nursing homes reveal that they are more concerned about the kindness of their caregivers, having their own space and their own friends, and the little details of their day-to-day life, than whether or not they have a valid Living Will or have decided about receiving cardiopulmonary resuscitation. In the nursing home, the little things count the most.[3]

Treatment Decisions

Because patients in nursing homes (who are usually chronically ill) sometimes become critically ill, many end-of-life treatment decisions must also be made.

Mrs. Lewis, eighty-two and an Alzheimer's patient, is experiencing kidney failure. For some time she has been noncommunicative, lying curled in a fetal position. Her family decides it would not be appropriate to subject her to dialysis or a kidney transplant, and she dies a rather peaceful death.

In the next room, Mrs. Peters, ninety-two but in reasonably good health, has developed a malignancy that could be treated by major surgery. Another alternative would be treatment by *irradiation* or *chemotherapy* that might extend her life but would likely cause significant unpleasant side-effects.

Mrs. Peters makes her own decision, in conjunction with her family and physician. She understands her condition, the treatment options, the likely outcome and possible risks of each option, and the likely result from no treatment.

She goes ahead with the surgery, with the understanding that if some secondary crisis occurs during the procedure, such as a heart attack, she does not desire to be resuscitated.

Now suppose Mrs. Peters survived the surgery, which was only moderately successful because of the extent of the tumor, but she develops pneumonia while still hospitalized. She has not recovered sufficiently to think clearly about the options. Should she be treated with antibiotics or not? If her respiratory function deteriorates, should she be transferred to the Intensive Care Unit for ventilator support?

The doctor explains to the family: "We need to weigh the benefit against the burden in this case, and take into consideration Mrs. Peters' prior wishes to refuse some forms of aggressive treatment. The benefit of antibiotics might be to cure the pneumonia and postpone her death for awhile."

"How long does she have, Doctor?" the daughter inquired. "I mean, if she gets over this pneumonia."

"Of course, we never can say precisely," the physician replied, "but considering her age and the type of malignancy, six months . . . maybe a year."

WISDOM OF THE AGES

Following is a beautiful but sobering passage in which we are reminded of our own inevitable physical deterioration and mortality:

> Remember your Creator in the days of your youth,
> before the days of trouble come and the years approach
> when you will say, "I find no pleasure in them"—before
> the sun and the light and the moon and the stars grow
> dark [the mind], and the clouds return after the rain;
> when the keepers of the house tremble [the hands],
> and the strong men stoop [bones], when the grinders
> cease because they are few [teeth], and those looking
> through the windows grow dim [eyes]; when the doors
> to the street are closed [lips] and the sound of grinding
> fades [hearing]; when men rise up at the sound of birds,
> but all their songs grow faint; when men are afraid of
> heights and of dangers in the streets [heart]; when the
> almond tree blossoms [white hair] and the grasshopper

drags himself along [kyphosis] and desire no longer is stirred [sexual function]. Then man goes to his eternal home and mourners go about the streets. Remember him—before the silver cord is severed [spinal cord], or the golden bowl [brain] is broken. (Ecclesiastes 12:1-6)

The time to serve God is in the days of our vigor and youth; later years may find us, as Ecclesiates describes, infirm and struggling to survive.

The realistic view of aging is that while many aged people are vigorous and productive, growing old also involves illness and loss. Bodily functions are impaired, family members and friends die, and chronic disease lingers.

Despite this reality, remembering that God has created us means that when long-term care decisions are required for someone, we must always keep the value of the person in focus. Decisions about Mrs. Henry, Mrs. Kaul, or Mrs. Peters are not so much about autonomy or costs or burdens versus benefits as they are about human beings who are unique and precious in God's sight.

Recognizing the Creator does not mean that all persons must be treated with all possible technology. Our life span is finite. Far better to improve the day-to-day aspects of patients' lives, to work with them to tailor treatment plans that honor their wishes, and to love and comfort them when the days of trouble come and the sun and the stars grow dark.

FOR DISCUSSION

Opening: Some group members may have struggled personally with the decision to bring an elderly parent into their home, or to put someone in a nursing home. Ask these members to share their experiences.

1. Ask each group member to say the first word that comes to mind when he or she thinks of a nursing home. Go around

again, and ask each one to describe a scene that comes to mind when he or she thinks of visiting a nursing home.

Are these words and images mostly positive, negative, or neutral? Discuss as a group why "nursing home" may seem to arouse more emotional response than some other health-care contexts; for instance, a hospital ward.

2. Have two group members read aloud the two parts of the brief "dialogue" involving the woman and her son (pages 124-125). Ask listeners to identify their emotional responses.

    Now expand this dialogue into a role-play by bringing in two other characters, the doctor and Nancy. In this role-play, the older woman is able to express herself verbally, too.

    After the role-play, a fifth actor will interview the other four, asking any questions that will draw out the emotions of such a difficult experience.

3. Tom (pages 126-128) has suggested that his mother's physician help deceive her into entering a health-care facility, in hopes that she will agree to stay there. He even goes so far as to suggest sedating her and moving her into such a facility while she is asleep.
    a. Do you think either or both of these options are ethical? Explain your answer, positive or negative.
    b. Considering Mrs. Henry's deteriorating condition, including bizarre behavior and paranoid thoughts, do you agree that something should be done, even against her will, for her own good? How would you approach this?

4. Discuss the relevance of these biblical texts to the question of paying for institutional long-term care for aging relatives:
    a. "If anyone does not provide for his relatives, and especially for his immediate family, he has denied the faith

and is worse than an unbeliever" (1 Timothy 5:8).

Does the Apostle Paul mean that adult children still have an obligation to provide financially for their parents? What if this would mean not being able to provide for their own children—for instance, providing a college education?

b. "Do not cast me away when I am old; do not forsake me when my strength is gone" (Psalm 71:9). Does this imply financial obligation, even if it should become a burden? What other obligations do you think are included?

c. Now integrate your thinking on the above passages with two other biblical texts:

"Honor your father and your mother" (Exodus 20:12).

"In everything, do to others what you would have them do to you, for this sums up the Law and the Prophets" (Matthew 7:12).

5. Mr. Kaul (page 128) learns that his good stewardship has caused his wife to be ineligible for financial assistance (until his resources are exhausted). He has come to you (his pastor) for advice. What alternative actions can you suggest?

6. As a member of Mrs. Peters' (pages 132-133) family, you have been asked by the doctor to decide whether or not to treat her pneumonia following the surgery. Canvass the group for their opinions and make your decision.

APPENDIX: DEMENTIA

Dementia is the general condition of widespread and irreversible loss of intellectual function. There are many causes, including brain tumors, brain injury, strokes, nutritional deficiencies, and degenerative diseases of the brain. The most common form of degeneration of brain function is Alzheimer's-type dementia; the basic underlying cause is as yet undetermined.

In the elderly, *Alzheimer's disease* is the fourth most common cause of death—following heart disease, cancer, and stroke.

The process of dementia is usually slow and progressive, with symptoms and signs appearing over a period of years. Occasionally the onset and course are more rapid. The earliest manifestation is usually impairment of recent memory followed by lack of initiative and inability to perform routine tasks. It may progress to reduced comprehension, lapses in social graces, and impaired judgment. There may be changes in mood and personality as well. In its later stages, there often is loss of ability to talk, walk, and control urination and defecation. Interest in eating and the ability to swallow are usually preserved. Death is most often caused by some complication of the bed-ridden state, such as pneumonia.

Certain reversible conditions may resemble dementia. Depression, reduced thyroid function, toxic reactions to medications, etc., may be found and corrected, restoring intellectual function. By definition, these conditions do not represent dementia. A person who is experiencing symptoms of dementia should have a thorough medical evaluation to find and reverse these other causes if possible.

NOTES:
1. Robert N. Butler, "Foreword," *Geriatric Medicine,* Christine K. Cassel and John R. Walsh, eds. (New York: Springer-Verlag, 1984), p. xv. See also White House Conference on Aging, final report, vol. 1 (Washington, DC: White House Conference on Aging, 1982); and Health and Public Policy Committee, American College of Physicians, "Long-Term Care of the Elderly," *Annals of Internal Medicine,* May 1984, 100:760-763.
2. Christine K. Cassel and Andrew L. Jameton, "Dementia in the Elderly: An Analysis of Medical Responsibility," *Annals of Internal Medicine,* June 1981, 94:802-807.
3. Joanne Lynn, ed., "Elderly Residents of Long-Term Care Facilities," *By No Extraordinary Means: The Choice to Forgo Life-Sustaining Food and Fluids* (Bloomington: Indiana University Press, 1986), p. 172.

Chapter Eight

A Non-Treatment
of Choice

Every time he makes a house call to visit Mrs. Williams, Dr. Nehls is profoundly impressed with her daughter's devotion and self-sacrifice. For nine years, Ruth has cared for her mother (the patient with Alzheimer's disease mentioned in chapter 1) as she has gradually deteriorated. Ruth and her family have made enormous sacrifices to care for Mrs. Williams, whose bed and medical supplies occupy a central area of the family's living room.

"SOMETIMES IT SEEMS SO FUTILE"

In the beginning, Mrs. Williams had been ambulatory and able to eat by herself. Eight years ago, after successful surgery for breast cancer, she began to decline. She took to bed. Her mental status deteriorated, and she began to require spoon-feeding. Then, one year later, she began having difficulty with spoon feeding, and a *feeding tube* was inserted.

Mrs. Williams has been hospitalized only on those occasions when liquid antibiotics failed to control her fevers, and she has not developed major aspiration pneumonias. Although she does not speak, she is aware of painful stimuli. She makes a low moaning sound when turned, and she seems to be aware of being bathed. Her skin is in good condition, indicating that she has been getting good nursing care. She receives weekly visits from a nurse, and Dr. Nehls comes to see her every two or three months.

During her mother's hospitalizations, Ruth has requested that Mrs. Williams not receive **cardiopulmonary resuscitation** (CPR) or intensive care unit treatment. Beyond this, however, Ruth has never expressed limits to her willingness to continue providing for her mother's basic needs until, as she put it, "the Lord takes Mother home."

Today, however, she asks Dr. Nehls to stay after his examination. "I've been thinking, Doctor," she begins slowly. "We've been wondering how long we can keep on with this."

She looked at the doctor and started to cry. "I'm sorry," she continued. "It's been so hard to know what's right, for her . . . for us. It's been so long, and sometimes it seems so futile. We've been immersed in Mother's dying for so long that we hardly remember what living is like. We can't afford institutional care, and we don't think that would be in her best interest, anyway. Will you help us decide what to do?"

Ten Years or Ten Days?

Ruth and her family have at least three possible options, according to Dr. Nehls:

1. Continue tube feeding and providing additional medical care when needed, which could go on for years. In fact, if Mrs. Williams survives until his next visit, it will already have been ten years since he first diagnosed her Alzheimer's disease.

2. Continue feeding, expecting that at some time Mrs.

Williams will develop another infection. If antibiotics were withheld, she might die at home not long thereafter.

3. Withdrawing her tube and withholding her feedings would result in her death within ten days to two weeks. "This is sometimes done in cases like this," the doctor added. "Many people are coming to see that feeding formula through a tube to someone who is without hope of recovery is a form of artificial medical treatment. In fact," he continued, "I sometimes wonder if it isn't less humane to force someone to continue existing in a state like your mother's instead of letting nature take its course." He paused, carefully studying Ruth's reaction. "Of course," he added, "whatever you decide, I will support you."

TO FEED OR TO WITHHOLD

This is one of the most basic but difficult ethical issues of the late twentieth century. One ethicist, in writing about the increasing number of chronically ill, marginally functioning elderly, said the denial of nutrition "could well become the nontreatment of choice."[1]

In answering Ruth's question, Dr. Nehls summarized a rather extensive, somewhat technical debate:[2]

"You Should Continue Feeding Mrs. Williams"

- Food and fluids are basic requirements of life, and therefore different than medical treatments. Artificially formulated food is still food, whether fed to infants or adults.
- Causing a person's death through withdrawal of food and fluids is similar to performing active euthanasia. If the intent is to bring death in ten to fourteen days, is it not more humane to bring death immediately, through injection?
- The provision of nutritional support is care, not technology, even though it uses technological means. Caring

for the helpless is basic human mercy, regardless of the recipient's age or quality of life, symbolizing a bottom-line human obligation. It is inhumane (and illogical) to decide not to feed someone because that person cannot feed himself.

"You May Stop Feeding Mrs. Williams"

- Withdrawal is acceptable when the situation is irreversible, death is imminent, or there is little hope of recovery of function. Continued feeding would be an indignity and a burden on patient and family, only prolonging the dying process.
- Nutritional support is not mandatory in all cases. Removing a feeding tube is no different than removing other technological support, such as a respirator, dialysis, or antibiotics.
- The symbolic or psychological value of feeding the totally dependent is not an important ethical/philosophical consideration.

TUBE FEEDING: PRO AND CON

MUST FEED BECAUSE	CAN STOP FEEDING BECAUSE
•Food is a basic requirement.	•Patient suffers irreversible disease.
•Withholding is equivalent to euthanasia.	•Tube feeding is an artificial means of support.
•Feeding means one cares.	•The value of feeding is merely symbolic.

LEGAL DIRECTIONS

The courts have fairly consistently considered tube feeding to be similar to respirators, dialysis machines, antibiotics, and chemotherapy; legal decisions have allowed the withdrawal of tube feeding by competent patients or their surrogates.[3]

When competent patients have requested the withdrawal

of their feeding tube, courts have decided that medically provided nourishment falls within the patient's right to refuse treatment. When patients are unable to state their wishes and their previous wishes are unknown, the courts have in most cases decided that withdrawal is acceptable in cases where tube feeding may cause unbearable suffering.

Increasingly, the courts are also deciding cases on a *quality-of-life* basis. For example, since it would be difficult to prove that patients with severe dementia are enduring "unbearable suffering" as a result of their tube feedings, legal scholar Roger Dworkin has said that in the case of Alzheimer's patient Claire Conroy, the court actually made a quality-of-life decision under the guise of "substituted judgment."[4]

While legal controversy continues in the area of withdrawal of nutritional support from incompetent patients, the trend is clearly toward legal sanction of this action based on a calculation of the perceived burdens and benefits to the patient or the perception of the patient's diminished quality of life. Despite these legal cases, sanctity of life considerations weigh in, generally, against the withdrawal of feeding tubes in Alzheimer's disease patients. In the case of a persistent vegetative state or irreversible coma, however, the absolute obligation to prolong life is clinically and ethically debatable.

PERSISTENT VEGETATIVE STATE (PVS)

When sixty-two-year-old Anna Thomas was admitted to the hospital, her physician, Dr. Susan Franklin, ordered her to be placed in the coronary care unit. She suspected that the woman's chest pain was from a heart attack. The following day, the patient suffered cardiac arrests. Although she regained consciousness after the first arrest, she remained unconscious after the second one.

"The *electroencephalogram*, or EEG, indicates Mrs. Thomas has experienced some brain damage due to lack of oxygen," the doctor explained to the family. "The neurologist predicts very little chance she will regain consciousness, and that if she does, severe neurologic disability is likely." The doctor paused, awaiting the reaction of her patient's family to this report.

"Can you tell us what you expect, Doctor?" the oldest son asked.

"Of course, we cannot be certain," the doctor continued, "but based on the neurologist's assessment, although your mother is breathing with the help of a respirator now, she will not require that long-term. However, Mrs. Thomas will probably remain in what is called a vegetative state, or irreversible coma. She might never recognize you or speak with you again. She will require feeding through a tube." The doctor paused again, thinking of the difficulties ahead for this family, and then added, "For now, we'll continue doing what we're doing, and we can all hope for improvements. We'll keep you fully informed, and you should feel free to ask any questions you have."

"I have one," Mrs. Thomas' daughter-in-law said. "How can I say this? We all love Mom—but are you saying that she could end up like Karen Anne Quinlan?"

UNCERTAINTY

In spite of modern technology and the data available on adults in coma, the prognosis for Mrs. Thomas is uncertain. She is not brain dead. She may end up in PVS and probably won't recover, but that is not one hundred percent certain. At least, it is much too soon after her cardiac arrests to be absolutely sure that her coma is permanent.

Dr. Franklin orders tube feeding for her patient. "It is on a trial basis," she explains to the family, "because we should at least give her a chance. This does not mean we will continue feeding her permanently, but there is enough uncertainty for now."

VULNERABILITY

Incompetent or institutionalized patients are vulnerable to withdrawal or withholding of care because their caregivers and families may decide that they are living "poor-quality lives." Because the survival of patients like Mrs. Thomas depends on medical orders, such considerations take on immense importance. But most quality-of-life judgments are quite subjective in nature, since many patients with neurologic illnesses who require life supports could be said to have "poor-quality lives." For this reason, decisions to discontinue feeding should probably not be made on quality-of-life considerations alone.

The Scriptures speak about the care of those who are defenseless and innocent: They are to be fed (Deuteronomy 14:29, Job 22:9) and protected, and we are to speak up for them (Isaiah 1:17).

CULPABILITY

Every time Dr. Franklin reviewed the issues of tube feeding (and they arose with more regularity than she preferred), two images kept coming into her mind: a photo album picture of her mother feeding her with a bottle, and a similar photo of herself with her own daughter.

She knew the philosophical arguments:

- "Withdrawing and withholding are ethically identical." *But they don't feel the same,* she thought.
- "Tube feeding is no different than any other medical procedure." *But somehow,* she continued the internal dialogue, *I know tube feeding is very different.*
- "Deaths resulting from discontinuance of tube feeding are equivalent to deaths from discontinuing dialysis or respirator."

  True, she thought. *But it's one thing to talk about discontinuing feeding someone. It's altogether different to actually do it, and to then have to watch the patient slowly die. How can you simply ignore the sense that you are somehow responsible?*

While a philosopher might say Dr. Franklin is being irrational here, the repugnance she feels about withdrawing nutritional support is natural. The debate over the withdrawal of tube feeding is new and, as yet, is unsettled. We think, however, that the withdrawal of tube feeding is permissible in some cases.

WHEN IS ENOUGH ENOUGH?

Ecclesiastes speaks about "a time to be born and a time to die." Prior to the use of feeding tubes, patients died when unable to take food offered to them by mouth. Suppose Anna Thomas lapsed into an irreversible coma. Would her feeding by tube—year after year—represent a futile endeavor to keep her body alive long past her "time to die"? Many would argue that it would, that somehow despite our desire to cherish and protect her life, Anna Thomas has lived past "her time." She will not wake up, but we will not let her die. Is this not a futile cycle?

The actual outcome of Anna Thomas' case is that she was allowed to die by withdrawal of her ventilator and blood pressure support medications. Dr. Franklin, after searching her own heart on the issue, would have been willing to withdraw the feeding tube as well, if her family had requested. But the patient died before this became an issue.

Many people consider the withholding or withdrawing of feeding tubes to be ethically permissible in cases of PVS, because they consider the patient to be suffering from an irreversible state of complete *cortical* brain damage. Despite our arguments against withdrawal of feeding tubes in general, and our concerns about the "slippery slope," we would seriously consider complying with the request of a well-intentioned family to withhold or withdraw tubes from their loved one if that person was in a state of clinical futility; that is, an irreversible unconsciousness in a persistent vegetative state.

However, our general practice is to continue feeding most patients despite the degree of neurological damage or disability, and we would consider each case individually and prayerfully.

Mrs. Williams Revisited

Although most of us would consider Mrs. Williams (who has had Alzheimer's disease for a decade) to be irreversibly ill, and none of us would personally wish to be in her situation, she is not brain dead. She is not in an irreversible coma either. The question is whether her daughter, Ruth, has the right to decide that it is in Mrs. Williams' best interest to be allowed to die through the withholding of food and fluids.

While Ruth has not requested the withdrawal of her mother's feeding tube, she has often spoken about how difficult it is to watch her deteriorate and how tragic this kind of end-of-life situation has been for both of them. During Dr. Nehls' most recent visit, he realized that he had not seen or heard mention of Ruth's husband during the past six months. He wondered. Stress like this often takes people beyond their breaking point. He made a mental note to gently inquire next time.

It is possible to argue that some patients might benefit from the withdrawal of feeding tubes—particularly those who are suffering a prolonged and painful death. There is an emerging consensus that tube feeding may be stopped at the request of competent patients or those who have an advance directive to that effect. But unless a demented patient states or previously has stated that he or she would not wish to be kept alive under the circumstances, there seems to be no patient-related justification, other than futility, for the withdrawal of feeding tubes.

This is an unresolved ethical issue on which there is no consensus. The problem, and the price, of a moral stance against withdrawal in these circumstances is that we will keep alive some patients who deep within their inaccessible minds want to die and are resentful that we do not let them die.[5]

The medical and philosophical tragedy of Alzheimer's disease, severe strokes, or PVS is that patients lose the ability to speak for themselves at the very time they most need to speak for themselves. The result is often, as in Mrs. Williams' case, an ethical problem regarding tube feeding. All of the alternatives are unfavorable or lamentable in some way.

First, Dr. Nehls could continue with care as he has in the past, giving Mrs. Williams food and antibiotics at the first sign of infection. But her dance toward death would seem on the most fundamental level to be a very slow and agonizing one for all involved.

Second, he could withhold her antibiotics and allow her to die from some future infection. But that may be no more humane than a death from feeding tube withdrawal. Of course, Dr. Nehls is just as uncertain about Mrs. Williams' wishes regarding withholding antibiotics as he is about her attitude toward withholding a feeding tube.

Third, he could withdraw her feeding tube, assuming that she would have wanted him to deny her food and water in her present condition. In order to take this direction, the patient's daughter would have to agree, both ethically and emotionally, with the withdrawal of nutritional support. If she and Dr. Nehls chose this option, they would have to admit making the decision based partly on futility or even on a quality-of-life judgment. If they chose this option, they would also have to come to terms with any legal, societal, or symbolic objections and handle any personal guilt involved.

In this case, we personally favor the first option—continuing tube feeding and antibiotics. But it would be intellectually dishonest to advocate this position without admitting we are troubled when thinking about Mrs. Williams. There are no easy answers here, and Christians can in good conscience disagree about tube feeding. We have talked with many Christians who would wish their feeding tube to be withheld or withdrawn if they themselves were to be in this situation.

FOR DISCUSSION

Opening: Have any group members who have experienced a tube-feeding decision in their family share the different aspects of their case, both the facts and how they feel (or felt) about the situation.

If no one has had such an experience, perhaps a nurse or doctor could talk about patients who have been fed by nasal tube or gastrostomy. Then have the group discuss their first impressions and reactions.

1. What would you do if you were Ruth or Dr. Nehls (pages 139-142)?

2. Do you think Anna Thomas' (pages 143-146) doctor would have been justified in withdrawing her feeding tube:
   a. at the request of her family?
   b. because of a Living Will?
   c. because of her poor quality of life?
   d. because the doctor and family decided continuing would be a futile fight against death?

3. Re-read Dr. Susan Franklin's internal dialogue with the philosopher-ethicists about tube feeding (pages 145-146). Which side do you think is the most rational? Which is the most humane? Which is the most biblical?

4. Do the Scriptures about caring for the defenseless and innocent really apply to the issue of tube feeding demented patients or those in irreversible coma? Read Deuteronomy 14:29, 24:17; Job 22:9; Isaiah 1:17; James 1:27. As a group,

develop timeless principles from these texts, and then discuss how they might be applied to withdrawing nutrition.

5. Do you think competent patients have a right to refuse tube feeding? On what basis:
   a. in secular ethics?
   b. in biblical ethics?

6. Discuss the importance of the following statement in terms of a tube-feeding decision in the case of Andy, a nineteen-year-old patient in his third year of PVS as the result of a motorcycle accident: "Feeding has symbolic importance in every society, including our own. At stake is our own understanding of our obligations toward a totally dependent person, whose needs and status some identify with the 'least of these' whom Jesus said we should love as part of loving Him." (See Matthew 25:40,45.)

NOTES:
1. Daniel Callahan, "On Feeding the Dying," *Hastings Center Report,* October 1983, 13:20-22.
2. See Patrick G. Derr, "Why Food and Fluids Can Never Be Denied," *Hastings Center Report,* February 1986, 16:28-30; John J. Paris, "When Burdens of Feeding Outweigh Benefits," *Hastings Center Report,* February 1986, 16:30-32; and Mark Siegler and Alan J. Weisbard, "Against the Emerging Stream: Should Fluids and Nutritional Support Be Discontinued?" *Archives of Internal Medicine,* January 1985, 145:129-131.
3. Robert Steinbrook and Bernard Lo, "Artificial Feeding—Solid Ground, Not a Slippery Slope," *New England Journal of Medicine,* February 4, 1988, 318:286-290.
4. Roger B. Dworkin, "Medicine, Ethics, and Law Reform," paper presented at the Center for Clinical Medical Ethics, February 25, 1987.
5. Daniel Callahan, *Setting Limits: Medical Goals in an Aging Society* (New York: Simon and Schuster, 1987).

Chapter Nine

Mercy Killing?

Jennie was only forty-eight when she found the breast lump. The surgeon had been hopeful, but the pathology report showed the cancer was very aggressive and had already spread to the lymph nodes. Radiation and chemotherapy were completed; everyone wished for the best, hoping and waiting.

Sadly, the wait wasn't long. In only a few months, Jennie developed back pain. The cause: spread of the breast cancer to her spine. The disease seemed to gallop through her bones, liver and lungs. She lost weight very rapidly, became depressed, and required large doses of morphine. The medication only partially relieved her severe pain. Any movement was excruciating.

It had been several weeks since she had smiled, desired food, or even enjoyed the brief visits of her loving children. Eventually her husband Sam asked, "Doctor, it's probably wrong to ask you this, but could you possibly give Jennie one large injection of morphine so that she won't suffer anymore? She's been in so much pain for so long. She just wants to get it over with."

Everyone was suffering: Jennie, Sam, the children, the nurses—yes, even the doctor suffered from his inability to control the patient's pain. All involved were ready for Jennie to die.

ACTIVE AND PASSIVE EUTHANASIA

The English word *euthanasia* is derived from a combination of Greek words: the adverb *eu* (well) and a form of the noun *thanatos* (death), usually meaning "a good death" (or an easy death). Euthanasia, in its classic usage, refers to mercy killing—the act of purposefully ending a human life with a motive of compassion. Most examples of mercy killing occur in the context of terminal cancer (e.g., a husband gives an overdose of sleeping pills to his wife who is suffering the excruciating pain of bone cancer). Euthanasia in humans is similar to a veterinarian giving a lethal injection to the severely injured or sick dog to "put it out of its misery." This is what Sam had in mind in his request to end Jennie's suffering: a deliberate act to bring about her rapid death. And this act of medical killing is what we mean throughout this chapter by the term *euthanasia*.

Sometimes, however, a distinction is made between *active* and *passive* euthanasia. Active euthanasia is defined as causing death directly by a deliberately fatal act, while passive euthanasia is defined as allowing a patient to die naturally by withholding or withdrawing treatment. We would say that withdrawing or withholding treatment or artificial means of life support in someone who is dying is not euthanasia at all—not even "passive" euthanasia—but acceptable, humane, and an often necessary part of everyday medical practice. Thus, *passive euthanasia* is not a helpful term; clarity of language is important when discussing this issue.

PLAYING GOD?

The ethical dilemmas raised by euthanasia are complex. As technology provides more and more ways of prolonging life, and as our society moves away from a Judeo-Christian value system, including its redemptive view of suffering, people are increasingly asking their physicians to end their lives. As absolutes, such as "Thou shalt not kill" from the Ten Commandments, and the Golden Rule, etc., diminish in importance, other rules become more powerful.

Self-determination (autonomy), for instance, affirms your "right to die" with dignity. Social justice (the greatest good for the greatest number) may further transform your "right to die" into a "duty to die" (if you're exhausting family or state resources). If it is your duty to die, is it then my duty as a physician (or family member) to help you fulfill your duty to die? It may even seem immoral of me to refuse. In fact, it may even become illegal to refuse. (If one calls evil good long enough, good will seem to become evil.)

Even sincere Christians, committed to the biblical truth that life is sacred and of inestimable value because man is made in God's image and He is sovereign, may find themselves requesting euthanasia when someone they love is dying and in great pain.

Sam (who loves God) requested that Jennie's life (he also loves Jennie) be ended by immediate overdose, which would be an illegal and immoral case of "active" euthanasia. But what if the physician, in administering enough narcotic to relieve the pain, should incidentally hasten her death through depressed respiration? Is this "double-effect euthanasia" more acceptable?

If you were Jennie, what would you want? Can it be the will of a loving God that His own children suffer terribly when there is medicine that would hasten a better death?

When ninety-five-year-old Mrs. Miller was admitted to the hospital suffering from a variety of illnesses and complications, her family requested "no heroics." The family was agreeable to providing normal sustenance (food and water), but was against providing other treatments that would only prolong her dying.

Could a loving family allow Mrs. Miller to die without intensive care? On what basis could the medical team cooperate with this family's wishes? Would withholding life-sustaining treatments be more justified if Mrs. Miller herself requested it? Is it playing God to withhold the treatment, or is it playing God to give such treatment to a patient who may be dying a natural death?

TO KILL OR TO LET DIE?

Modern medical technology has developed remarkable means to prolong our living—and our dying. There is almost always something more that could be done. So someone has to decide when enough has already been done; when it is time to let the patient die. In recent years, that decision has fallen to the courts, with one ruling amplifying another as the legal system has tried to grapple with these relatively new life-and-death decisions.

For example, in the case of *Rudolpho Torres*, the Minnesota Supreme Court ruled that the respirator sustaining his life could be disconnected because, as one writer put it, "Mr. Torres may well have wished to avoid . . . the ultimate horror not of death but the possibility of being maintained in limbo, in a sterile room, by machines controlled by strangers."[1]

Increasingly, the courts have been allowing the withdrawal or withholding of life supports (including nutrition and hydration), in cases broader than those where patients are terminally ill or in unrelenting pain. Although the trend is toward a broader interpretation of the right to refuse treatment, there is still a sharp division of legal, ethical, and medical opinion on this issue.

For committed Christians, what in theory may seem rather

black and white can become rather gray in practice. When
eighty-six-year-old Grandma Davis developed breast cancer,
the family and doctor decided against aggressive chemotherapy.
They favored less stressful hormonal treatment, knowing that
while chemotherapy might prolong her life, it could also make
her life miserable because she might not understand the reason for the treatment and she would be subjected to numerous
injections, infusions, blood draws, side effects, etc. Less aggressive treatment would mean a shorter but more peaceful life. As
Grandma's death grew near, the doctor and family decided not
to force feed her or treat her pneumonia with antibiotics or a
ventilator. She died quietly at home a few hours after receiving
a dose of pain medication, and she appeared to be comfortable
and pain-free at the very end.

Grandma Davis' death was a "good death," if any death
can be called good. It was certainly a better death than many
others have experienced from cancer. But was it euthanasia?
Were the decisions that were made good decisions? Because
Grandma could not make her own decisions, the family had
to make them for her. They chose not to aggressively treat
her disease, for they didn't wish to delay the inevitable. In the
end, they chose not to force-feed her, because they viewed the
extension of her life a few more hours or days as futile. Her
physician agreed.

So Grandma Davis' death was not a case of euthanasia.
Yes, there was that injection, given just hours before her death,
to ease her struggle to breathe. But in euthanasia there is rapid
and intentional death, and if the doctor had chosen the timing
of death rather than the Lord, Grandma Davis might have been
denied that sense of transcendent peace when she died.

We wanted to present Grandma Davis' case to make it
clear that she was not killed; she died. This is an important
point, because some ethicists argue that there is no difference
between passive and active euthanasia.[2] This sort of confusion
muddles the real issues of medical killing. The result is that
euthanasia, which is evil, can be classified as acceptable if it

is allowed to be redefined, since it is totally acceptable to let Grandma Davis die as she did. If a term like *passive eutha-nasia* is acceptable today, it becomes much easier to accept the practice of *active euthanasia* tomorrow.

THE MODERN EUTHANASIA MOVEMENT

The modern euthanasia movement in the West—in the Netherlands and the United States—has been characterized thus far by emphasis on the voluntary consent of the patient who would request to be killed. Physicians in the Netherlands perform active euthanasia at the patient's request. While euthanasia is illegal in the Netherlands, it is sanctioned by society and physicians are rarely prosecuted. Estimates are that Dutch physicians kill five to eight thousand patients per year.[3] (This would extrapolate to 80 to 130 thousand with comparable practice in the United States.)

Over the several years that this has been happening in Holland, an average of eleven cases a year have been investigated by public prosecutors. In those few cases brought to trial, the court has found the physician guilty, but has not imposed punishment. Sometimes on appeal a court has overturned the verdict on the grounds that the doctor acted out of "higher necessity."

Dutch physicians who perform euthanasia inject patients with fatal doses of phenobarbital and curare. The guidelines of the Royal Dutch Medical Association for performing euthanasia are listed below.[4]

Euthanasia in Holland: "Guidelines"

1. The performance of euthanasia actions should rest upon voluntariness.
2. The patient should be experiencing unacceptable and prospectless suffering which can no longer be made bearable.

3. The patient's longing for death should be durable and well-considered.
4. The case should be discussed with colleagues.
5. Euthanasia should be performed in a medically pharmacologically justified way.
6. Death certificates should not be falsified (e.g., "pneumonia") but should state that euthanasia was performed.

The CBS televised documentary "The Last Right" presented a chilling glimpse of euthanasia in Holland. One daughter rather casually described her mother's death by injection. The mother, who had terminal cancer, had spelled out in advance exactly what she wanted: "I'm willing to go on as long as possible," she said, "but the minute I can't function any more, and I'll be reduced to something that's kept alive, I just don't want that. The minute I say, 'This is enough,' that is the moment I want to die." And so she died, her final words being, "Yes, I want it to happen," and "It's so nice to see you all again. Bye-bye," and "Please do it now."

Shortly after the fatal dose, the daughter was reassuring her mother, saying, "It will be all over now. Things are going the way you wanted." The physician said rather matter-of-factly to the daughter, "Well, you can stop talking, you know. She's dead."[5]

Euthanasia in the United States
The "Humane and Dignified Death Act" (a proposed addition to California Civil Code) was sponsored by right-to-die advocates. The proposal, which on the first round failed to obtain enough signatures to appear on the ballot, would have allowed terminal patients to request that their doctors give them lethal injections. The Humane and Dignified Death Act makes no ethical distinction between withdrawing and withholding life-sustaining treatment and performing active euthanasia: "Any declarant may execute a directive directing the withholding or

withdrawal of life-sustaining procedures or administering aid in dying . . . the directive must be signed by the declarant in the presence of two witnesses."

Because the patients are competent, the proponents argue, and the request is totally voluntary, the physician is not culpable. The physician is not deciding who should be killed or making quality-of-life judgments; rather, he or she is assisting a suicide. Again, the blurring: between suicide, assisted suicide, withdrawal or withholding of medical treatment, and active euthanasia by lethal injection. This sort of proposal is being put forth in other states. How will voters begin to sort out these differences, when even those who study and debate these issues every day have mixed them all together?

Trying to Stem the Tide

A growing number of secular writers on the topic do not appeal to the rightness or wrongness of euthanasia, but state that it should not be legalized because of *the bad consequences* of such a change in our society. Such bad consequences are:

- *Abuse.* Once it is considered right to end someone's life on request, it will be much easier to presume a "request" from others (the demented, comatose, etc.).
- *Error.* The inherent uncertainties in medicine will cause some to die unnecessarily.
- *Slippery slope.* Once society accepts voluntary euthanasia, it can be predicted that very quickly allowance will have to be made for those who are unable to speak for themselves.
- *Distrust.* If the patient knows his doctor is allowed to kill him, there will be an erosion of the traditional trust between patient and doctor.
- *Coercion.* Elderly, handicapped, and dying people may feel subtly or directly encouraged to request their legal option of euthanasia.

These consequential arguments against euthanasia may be sufficiently convincing for some, but they cannot answer the basic question, "Is euthanasia wrong?"

AUTONOMY'S ULTIMATE ACT?

Proponents of euthanasia believe that the request from a competent person to be killed is the ultimate autonomous act. Whether their motivation is relief of suffering, or reduction of the burden on their family or society, they say they are exercising free choice over their destiny. They claim they are taking charge and are deciding what is best for themselves.

But assisted suicide or active-voluntary euthanasia are not truly autonomous acts, since each involves at least one other individual—an individual who remains behind to struggle with issues of responsibility, morality, guilt, and remorse.

We, the People

Since public opinion polls reveal that euthanasia would be acceptable to many in our society, should euthanasia be legalized in the United States? In this democracy, can the state demonstrate a compelling reason for withholding what the people want? Is freedom to choose the moment of death an important aspect of liberty? Is the choice to actively end one's own life inherently wrong?

The U.S. Declaration of Independence states that the inalienable human rights are "life, liberty and the pursuit of happiness." The order in which these are listed is not coincidental. Life is fundamental and is necessary in order to achieve liberty or happiness. A person's freedom to choose (liberty) is by necessity dependent on having life itself. Even a person living in suffering (i.e., without happiness) still has some choices (e.g., the choices about treatment, coping, relationships, and eternal questions).

Those people who maintain that euthanasia should be allowed in those cases where there is intolerable suffering are saying, in essence, that the immediate absence of suffering is a higher good than liberty or life.

"THOU SHALT NOT MURDER"

Prohibition of the direct taking of human life, except in self-defense or in the defense of others, has been a central tenet of Judeo-Christian tradition and teaching. This is based on the Sixth Commandment, "Thou shall not kill [murder]" (Deuteronomy 5:17, KJV). Human life is a gift of our sovereign God, who alone is entitled to determine when and how an individual life will end.

The ethics and tradition of medicine have emphasized the preservation of human life and repudiated the direct taking of life. The Hippocratic Oath states very clearly, "I will not administer poison to anyone when requested nor make a suggestion to that effect." This prohibition is reiterated by the judicial council of the American Medical Association: "The intentional termination of the life of one human being by another—mercy killing—is contrary to that for which the medical profession stands and is contrary to the policy of the AMA."[6]

Judeo-Christian tradition teaches that it is wrong for one person to kill another, even out of mercy. Medical tradition teaches the same thing. Many modern thinkers, without appealing to either of these traditions, believe it is wrong because of the consequences of medical killing. They reason that such an act is simply not part of the doctor's job description, because killing patients goes against several thousands of years of medical ethics.

The effects of widespread euthanasia on the doctor-patient relationship are predictable and negative in the long run. Margaret Mead reported that in societies where doctors actively kill patients, the sick are apprehensive. What will their doctor do to them? History demonstrates that physicians may act quickly and unilaterally to bring patients' lives to an end.

The outcome of the Netherlands' experience with active

euthansia is still too early to assess: their culture is very different from ours. Promoting euthanasia in a rapidly aging, cost-conscious society like ours may present policy problems. Our medical system is too fragmented and is undergoing too much economic and structural upheaval to make euthanasia a prudent policy choice. Finally, the euthanasia movement would largely ignore the great progress made in pain control and in compassionate hospice care. Why not correctly care for the dying instead of killing them?

But what if the consequences seem to be entirely personal, as in suicide? What if a person kills himself or herself because he or she cannot tolerate life as it is? Is that wrong as well?

SUICIDE

Some ancient societies (e.g., ancient Greece) condoned and even encouraged suicide. This was usually justified philosophically on the basis of man's radical freedom. Some modern cultures still view suicide as acceptable; in Japan, taking one's own life has been viewed as a matter of honor.

In Anglo-American society, suicide has long been illegal. Suicides were punished by burial in unconsecrated ground, and acts of attempted suicides were considered felonies. In the United States, all states have now decriminalized suicide itself, but in most states the law still forbids assisting in a suicide. Evidence that a person is a clear danger to himself or herself is grounds for involuntary psychiatric commitment proceedings; again, the inalienable human right of life goes before other rights.

The Bible has no explicit prohibition against suicide. Most Bible scholars believe that the Sixth Commandment applies to self-murder as well. Several examples of suicide are recorded in Scripture: Saul and his armor-bearer (1 Samuel 31:4-5), Ahithophel (2 Samuel 17:23), Zimri (1 Kings 16:18), Judas (Matthew 27:5). Most commentators believe that suicide is condemned by inference in these instances. According to Augustine, even Samson's heroic suicide was evil (Judges 16:29-30).

Modern thought often ignores the teachings of religions, traditions, and cultures. Man is portrayed as the center of the universe, yesterday's values are obsolete, and self-determination is the primary principle. It is this philosophy that is behind the current effort to help people commit suicide and legalize euthanasia. One example of this effort is the publication by the Hemlock Society of a book entitled *Let Me Die Before I Wake,* a practical guide on how to successfully take one's life or assist another in suicide. Another book has been published by a woman who describes how she helped her mother commit suicide.

People who support suicide and/or euthanasia appeal to compassion for the dying and a person's right to final self-determination. However, most terminally ill people do not choose suicide; if they do, it is out of desperation and despair. They take their own lives because they can no longer tolerate the physical or emotional suffering they are experiencing. "I am in too much pain. I am no use to anyone. I cannot live this way." Like Jennie, they just want to die.

BEYOND THE PAIN TO MEANING

In their pain, suicide and euthanasia victims ignore an even more basic question: Is there any meaning or purpose to suffering? Is there really any alternative to pain and suffering? Viktor Frankl, Austrian psychiatrist imprisoned in Auschwitz for three years, says "Suffering ceases to be suffering in some way at the moment it finds meaning."[7] Nietzsche said, "He who has a *why* to live can bear almost any *how.*"[8]

Dr. Paul Brand, noted Christian surgeon, believes there is a purpose for physical pain in our material world. He found that his leprosy patients were injuring themselves because they lacked pain sensation in their hands and feet. He tried to develop an artificial pain system for his patients, but his attempts were unsuccessful because the patients always turned off or ignored the artificial pain system. They didn't understand their need for pain. He concluded that pain sensation is a marvel, a bioengineering masterpiece of warning and protection. Even if we don't want it, pain is necessary.[9]

But suffering is more than just physical pain. Suffering includes emotional pain (grief), social pain (loneliness), financial pain (poverty), and spiritual pain (guilt). A person may choose suicide or request euthanasia for any one or a combination of these components of "total pain."

We do not mean to glorify suffering. On the contrary, according to the biblical world view, painful toil (for Adam) and increased pains in childbearing (for Eve) are a part of the curse that God imposed on human beings in the material world as a result of rebellion (Genesis 3:16-17). These painful experiences were in addition to the more basic spiritual pain of a fractured relationship with the Creator.

Christians can believe and rejoice that in the Kingdom, "There will be no more death or mourning or crying or pain, for the old order of things has passed away" (Revelation 21:4). But we are still inhabitants of this fallen world—the "old order of things." If God promised us a pain-free existence on earth as a reward for following Him, people would choose to be "believers" for the wrong reason. He wants us to choose Him freely, not for what we can get out of Him. And we can't get out of pain anyway. It happens.

But what is the purpose of a specific pain in a specific person at a specific time? Is there a purpose, or is God just capricious?

Sometimes pain is corrective. God uses it to get our attention and make us realize we are walking our own path instead of His way: "But you have planted wickedness, you have reaped evil, you have eaten the fruit of deception. Because you have depended on your own strength . . ." (Hosea 10:13).

Other times, pain is meant to help us grow and develop: "And the God of all grace, who called you to his eternal glory in Christ, after you have suffered a little while, will himself restore you and make you strong, firm and steadfast" (1 Peter 5:10).

God sometimes allows suffering for His glorification. The disciples asked Jesus if it was the sin of the blind man or that of his parents that was the cause of his affliction. Jesus responded, "Neither this man nor his parents sinned . . . but this happened so that the work of God might be displayed in his life" (John 9:3).

Man's correction, man's development, or God's glorification. One, two, three purposes for pain; sounds nice and pat. But we know the other reasons are often hidden from us. Consider Jennie, a forty-eight-year-old woman dying of breast cancer in the prime of her life. Why? We know that the answer isn't always straightforward. We are not always able to see the big picture. We are reminded in Deuteronomy 29:29, "The secret things belong to the LORD our God, but the things revealed belong to us."[10]

In the past, pain was accepted as a part of life; not glorified, but accepted. Today's attitude is more frequently that all pain must be stopped and eliminated. When someone is suffering and sees no meaning or purpose, and no hope for improvement, despair is the result. This can be the path to suicide attempts or requests for euthanasia.

OUR RESPONSE

What should be our response to someone who pleads, "I can't stand the suffering! Kill me or help me kill myself!"? There are two valid responses, and both should be made available.

One response is a *hospice* answer: "I can't kill you, but I can still help you. Because I won't kill you, I have a great moral responsibility to ease your suffering. Let me treat your pain (medically) as effectively as I can; let me hold your hand; let me help you address your emotional, financial, and spiritual needs. Let me be your friend, so that when you die you will not die alone." Hospice has demonstrated that physicians should be better educated about pain management and better equipped to treat pain effectively. More than ninety-five percent of cancer patients can be kept virtually pain free if they are given adequate doses of pain medication at appropriate intervals.

The other response is to try to help the person gain insight into his or her suffering, to find some meaning in the plight; to help the sufferer see that there is a sovereign, loving God who has allowed this situation for His purpose—a purpose that we may or may not be able to discern. This response involves letting God's love shine through us. Second Corinthians 1:3-4 reveals that He is our example: "The God of all comfort, who comforts us in all our troubles, so that we can comfort those in any trouble with the comfort we ourselves have received from God."

Above all, we can offer hope—the hope that pain is temporary, that glory is forever, that Heaven is free of suffering and tears. And we can be with those who suffer, pray with them, and love them.

FOR DISCUSSION

Opening: Ask group members to briefly share any experiences they have had with euthanasia or suicide.

1. Using Jennie's case (pages 151-152), try to define the main issues for the different persons who may be drawn into this discussion.
   a. For the person/patient:
   b. For the family/friends:
   c. For the doctor/medical team:
   d. For the pastor/church:

2. a. If you were dying and in great pain, what do you think you would really want for yourself?

b. If you were in a coma, with no hope of recovery, would you want to be kept alive?

c. In either situation, would you want your doctor to have the freedom to:

___ end your life directly, if the pain became unbearable?

___ treat the pain aggressively, even if it meant that you might die earlier of a secondary effect?

___ hasten your death by withdrawing or withholding treatment?

___ hasten your death by withholding food and water?

d. To what degree do biblical principles affect your choices?

3. One argument for legalizing euthanasia is that the greatest fear of modern man is that through illness or accident we may spend our last days (or even years) in a dehumanized state of suspended animation, kept alive by artificial means in a sterile environment by people we don't know.

Compare and prioritize these death-related fears, from greatest to least:

___ death itself

___ dying slowly, but not in pain

___ dying slowly, in great pain

___ abandonment/isolation while dying

___ dying in alienation from God

___ dying without a sense of fulfillment or meaning

___ being killed by someone else

___ the possibility of killing myself

4. Below are two of the Apostle Paul's comments to the Corinthian Christians, which can be related to euthanasia issues:

a. "You are not your own; you were bought at a price. Therefore honor God with your body" (1 Corinthians 6:19-20).

Although the context here is motivation for shunning immorality, the principle is that we are to honor God with the way we use our body, because He owns us. Discuss the difference between this idea and the modern assertion of an autonomy so radical that it includes the right to take my own life.

b. "Therefore we do not lose heart. Though outwardly we are wasting away, yet inwardly we are being renewed day by day. For our light and momentary troubles are achieving for us an eternal glory that far outweighs them all. So we fix our eyes not on what is seen, but on what is unseen. For what is seen is temporary, but what is unseen is eternal" (2 Corinthians 4:16-18).

How can the hope that springs from knowing God become a motivation to embrace whatever path He has set before us, even if this includes great suffering?

NOTES:
1. Beth Spring and Ed Larson, *Euthanasia* (Portland, OR: Multnomah Press, 1988).
2. See James Rachels, *The End of Life: Uthanasia and Morality* (New York: Oxford University Press, 1986).
3. Gregory E. Pence, "Do Not Go Slowly into that Dark Night: Mercy Killing in Holland," *American Journal of Medicine,* January 1988, 84:139-141.
4. Central Committee of the Royal Dutch Medical Association, "Vision on Euthanasia," *Medical Contact,* 1984, 39:990-998.
5. CBS/Broadcast Group, *60 Minutes* transcript, August 21, 1988, p. 11.
6. "Withholding or Withdrawing Life-Prolonging Treatment," *Current Opinions of the Council on Ethical and Judicial Affairs of the AMA—1986* (Chicago: American Medical Association, 1986).
7. Viktor Frankl, *Man's Search for Meaning* (New York: Pocket Books, 1963).
8. Frankl, p. 164.
9. Philip Yancey, *Where Is God When It Hurts?* (Grand Rapids, MI: Zondervan, 1977).
10. The question of pain/suffering has been addressed by many writers and is beyond the scope of our book, although it is a crucial consideration. We recommend these books for further study: C. S. Lewis, *The Problem of Pain* (New York: Macmillan, 1962); Peter Kreeft, *Making Sense Out of Suffering* (Ann Arbor, MI: Servant Books, 1986); David Biebel, *If God Is So Good, Why Do I Hurt So Bad?* (Colorado Springs, CO: NavPress, 1989); Philip Yancey, *Where Is God When It Hurts?* (Grand Rapids, MI: Zondervan, 1977); and Edith Schaeffer, *Affliction* (Toronto, ON, Canada: Welch, 1973).

Chapter Ten

When It's Only
a Matter of Time

She's asking me to decide when Sally will die, Jim thought, trying to focus on what the doctor was saying, listening with his ears but struggling with his heart. *After fifty-three years of marriage, it comes to this. How can I make that kind of decision? How can anyone make that kind of decision?*

"There's nothing more that can be done about the cancer," Dr. Shaw continued. "Sally's condition is rapidly deteriorating, as you know. It's really only a matter of time." She paused, measuring Jim's reaction before continuing.

Jim nodded, his voice wavering with emotion. "I know."

"We still have several options," the doctor said. "We can continue intravenous fluids, and she will linger on awhile—perhaps two or three weeks—or we can discontinue the fluids, in which case she will probably die within several days. Either direction is morally acceptable, in my opinion."

Jim nodded again, but inside he knew that none of it was

emotionally acceptable. In the space of just a few months, his life—their life together—had been forever shattered. His mind raced through the scenes etched like snapshots in his memory. Sally had fallen, coming out of church on Christmas Eve, and broken her hip. X-rays revealed that a tumor had invaded and weakened the bone. Then the surgery, the radiation, the mixture of hope and then despair, as it gradually became clear the cancer was spreading. In a way, that was the only thing that was clear in the whole experience.

Just before she left, Dr. Shaw reminded Jim that two days earlier while she was making morning rounds, Sally stirred briefly from her unconscious state long enough to say, "I wish they would stop all this." Then she drifted off again.

"Dear God, what should I do?" Jim struggled for words as he prayed later that night. "Dr. Shaw would like a decision in the next day or two. Why does a decision have to be made? Can't we just let nature take its course? And why is it my decision? Can't the doctor decide? Can't Sally help? Can't somebody help? Dear God, what should I do?"

Only a few years ago, Sally's physician might not have involved Jim in the decision. The gradual change from the paternalistic approach that physicians used to use to the current shared decision-making process places greater requirements on the physician as he or she tries to balance the principles of truth-telling, the duty to do no harm, and the patient's right to self-determination.

This balancing requires a careful and sensitive telling of the truth. Dame Cecily Saunders, the founder of the hospice movement in Britain, wrote, "The alternatives are not merely silence, bland denial or stark fatal truth. There are many different truths just as there are many ways of imparting them. We have to learn to give the one the individual needs at that moment in the simplest and kindest way we can offer it."[1]

This sounds like the scriptural admonition about "speaking the truth in love" (Ephesians 4:15), a delicate enough proposition when the issues are not life and death. In this case,

Dr. Shaw had tried to be sensitive to Jim's feelings as she explained Sally's terminal situation and the options available.

After prayerful consideration, which included input from family members and their pastor, Jim called Dr. Shaw to let her know that they had a sense of peace about not extending Sally's struggle any longer than necessary. The doctor had their permission to discontinue the intravenous treatment. Sally was given oral fluids and mouth care as tolerated. She died several days later of cancer and its complications.

"YOU HAVE THE POWER"

Sometimes the patient himself makes the decision to discontinue treatment.

Sitting up in the hospital bed, struggling for air despite a high flow of oxygen, Mrs. Hanson had said to the doctor on several occasions, "You have the power . . . ," but she was unable to complete the thought. Only after playing "twenty questions" did the doctor understand: Mrs. Hanson wanted to die soon. She didn't want any more active therapy. No more removal of the fluid around her lung. No more chemotherapy. No more transfusions.

Following her surgery for uterine cancer fifteen months earlier, Mrs. Hanson, a sixty-four-year-old widow, made a good initial recovery. But as the malignancy spread to her chest, Mrs. Hanson and her physician had a frank discussion about the likelihood of this disease taking her life.

In the intervening months, Mrs. Hanson had slowly given away many of her family heirlooms. She had written cheerful letters of farewell to friends and family. She had asked the doctor to pray for grace and comfort for her as she finished her earthly life.

Now she wanted the doctor to pray with her again. For the first time in his practice, he asked a patient, "Do you want me to pray for you to die?" She nodded vigorously, and as the doctor held her hand, he prayed that she would die.

The doctor then began wrestling with the possibilities: "If I give Mrs. Hanson more transfusions and continue to remove her chest fluid, she may live several more days, even two weeks.

"If I follow her request, she will die sooner. But she will die very short of breath—not a pleasant way to spend her last hours. I could give her more morphine which will relieve some of her pain and breathlessness, but that might in fact hasten her death by suppressing her respirations.

"She's right. In a way, under God I do have the power. I have the power to control when and in what state she dies. It's an awesome power, and a grave responsibility—one that must be controlled and directed by trustworthy guiding principles."

A TIME TO DIE—BUT WHEN?

Everyone will die, as the Scriptures remind us: "There is a time for everything, and a season for every activity under heaven: a time to be born and a time to die" (Ecclesiastes 3:1-2).

However, over the millenia, the details have changed. Even two generations ago most people with terminal illnesses died at home, wearing their own pajamas, looking at familiar wallpaper, cared for by family and friends. Their treatment was "tender loving care," plus some morphine for the pain.

Today in North America, seventy percent of people die in health-care institutions, wearing hospital gowns, looking at sterile walls, attended by strangers. Many medical and surgical therapies are available—most involving insertion of tubes accompanied by intrusive gadgets that buzz, beep, and whir.

The hospice movement, which began in Britain and came to North America in the early 1970s, has done much to re-humanize the dying process. With the shift in emphasis from curing to caring and living each day until death, more people are spending a greater percentage of their last weeks at home rather than in the hospital, often with the help of volunteers who serve as surrogate family members. Hospice writers have reminded those in the medical profession that patients who are dying need emotional, social, financial, and spiritual support as well as physical attention. Still, most patients die in hospitals rather than at home.

The needs of family members are also important. They suffer, too, as they watch loved ones go through the dying process. Most deaths are anticipated and happen slowly over a period of days, weeks, or months. However, even when death is inevitable, there is usually a range of treatment options from aggressive palliation (with the goal being to slow disease process) to aggressive symptom control (with the goal being to comfort the patient).

The decision is not a question of treatment versus non-treatment, but a problem of defining the goals of treatment and deciding which are appropriate for a particular patient at a particular time. With today's wide range of treatment options, there is almost always "something more" that can be done to postpone death. There can be another blood transfusion, more intravenous fluids, correction of salt and water imbalance, another operation, more radiation, etc. The timing of death becomes a matter of choice.

If people have some measure of control over the time of death, does this contradict the Scripture's affirmation that God is sovereign? (See 1 Chronicles 29:11-12.) Are we "playing God" when we hasten or postpone death? The Lord says, "I put to death and I bring to life, I have wounded and I will heal, and no one can deliver out of my hand" (Deuteronomy 32:39).

God *is* sovereign and *is* in control. He has given people free will to live in His created world within the laws of nature He has established. He has also given us the capacity to develop and use scientific techniques that extend life.

Every time a physician treats an infection with an antibiotic, the course of life may be altered. Is this "playing God"? No, for if God has allowed us to develop medical skills, then we are stewards of these skills and are responsible to Him for how we use them. In using them we must not violate His precepts.

God, of course, is not restricted to operating within the laws of nature or science. He created the laws, and He has the power to decide in certain instances to miraculously work above and beyond them. This can account for the occasional unexpected "spontaneous remission" of a seemingly terminal illness.

Faced with a range of treatment choices, however, the patient and physician must make some practical decisions based on the possible advantages and disadvantages of each option. These decisions usually take into consideration the implications for the patient, the family, and occasionally society also. Making the decisions involves communication, understanding, and the use of reason. As professor Howard Hendricks of Dallas Theological Seminary pointed out in one of his sermons, "The passage says we shouldn't *lean* on our own understanding, but [God] never says don't *use* it!"

During the dying process, the patient's ability to make decisions may be clouded by the disease itself, by pain, or by drugs given to relieve pain. When this happens, the physician must rely on the patient's previously spoken wishes or on written advance directives. If there is no clear expression of the patient's desire, the physician must turn to a surrogate for assistance with decisions.

Sometimes physicians may be reluctant to give less than maximal treatment. They rightly view their primary mission as treating disease and postponing death, and feel they are giving up if they don't do what is possible. Or they may have less defensible reasons: the neurotic fear of failure or the fear of being sued for malpractice if survivors are distressed that "not everything was done." But doctors need to remember that their primary mission is caring for patients along with fighting disease. Do they really have the right to prescribe a lingering death if the patient chooses only comfort measures?

Many people talk about a "right to die." What is actually meant by this phrase is that patients have a right to refuse treatment, a right which is optional. The right to refuse treatment, and then die, should not be confused with the *duty* to refuse treatment or the *duty* to die. If the person has a duty to die, it would seem a short step to implying a *duty* to help someone die (see Chapter Nine). A patient has the right to decline treatment, even life-saving treatment, and if he or she chooses to refuse a treatment, then the doctor or the patient's family should not force treatment on the patient.

THE DILEMMAS OF CPR

For the first time since their six-year-old son Eddie had become ill three months earlier, Mr. and Mrs. Johnson were about to go out for a quiet dinner together, thanks to the nursing care that had been arranged. The stress of the past few weeks had been exhausting, and they wondered what would happen to Eddie. Since their first son had died of a similar rare disorder, they feared Eddie would die, too. There was also another fear—that Eddie would survive but never recover from the brain injury which had left him nearly helpless.

As the Johnsons prepared to leave, they were caught off guard by the nurse's question: "If something should happen to Eddie while you're out, would you want me to try to bring him back?"

The Johnsons looked at each other. Their first son had slipped away suddenly, to everyone's surprise, about five weeks after the illness began. Perhaps the same thing might happen again. Why fight it? If this was how it was supposed to end, wouldn't it be better to let it end instead of making the agony last longer than necessary?

The nurse gave them a form which they signed, authorizing her not to try to revive Eddie if he should have such a crisis while they were gone.

Cardiopulmonary resuscitation (CPR) is a therapy that has saved many lives but also has created new dilemmas. Prior to the early 1960s, death was declared when the patient stopped breathing or the heart stopped beating. This was a fairly precise point in time that made the determination of death relatively easy. Then, with the development of cardiac surgery, it was learned that cessation of a heartbeat was merely an electrical and mechanical event that could be reversed.

Is death reversible? Not really. It is just that all the cells of the body don't die the instant the heart stops. If the heart is re-started before other body tissues begin to deteriorate, the patient may be successfully resuscitated.

Development of artificial respiration and external cardiac massage made it possible to artificially maintain breathing and circulation while simultaneously attempting to chemically or electrically revive the heart. This procedure, usually referred to as CPR, has become very sophisticated and standardized. The resuscitation process can go on for an hour or even longer, depending on whether the heart resumes function. However, if CPR is going to be successful, the patient's heart will usually resume functioning after only a few minutes. If CPR is not successful, the patient is declared dead.

CPR was first developed for use only on victims of near-drowning or electrocution. Now it is employed widely in hospitals. In addition, many members of the general public have learned how to perform CPR. This emergency treatment is sometimes initiated by bystanders when someone collapses at home, in a restaurant, or on the street.

CPR is attempted in one third of cardiac arrests with these results:

> If one hundred hospital patients receive CPR,
> seventy will die despite the attempt;
> thirty will survive the attempt;
> twenty of the thirty initial survivors will die before they
>   leave the hospital;
> six of the ten final survivors will be alive five years later.[2]

It is crucial that patients and families realize that CPR is routine in hospitals, regardless of the patient's condition, unless there is a specific order to the contrary. The specific order against CPR ("Do Not Resuscitate," DNR) is only about fourteen years old, but it is widely and effectively used. Two-thirds of hospitalized patients or their families decide to forego resuscitation. The DNR order requires the consent of the patient or surrogate. This is consistent with the concept that a patient may decide to forego life-sustaining therapy—and CPR is the ultimate form of life-sustaining therapy. When such an order is written, it does not mean that the patient is abandoned; necessary treatments should still be provided.

Of all body tissues, brain cells are the most delicate; they begin to die after about four minutes without oxygen. Once damaged, brain tissue heals very poorly. If the brain receives insufficient oxygen during attempted resuscitation, part or all of the brain may be damaged, but the remainder of the body may survive. Sometimes only one localized area of brain tissue is damaged, and on awakening the patient appears to have had a stroke. This can be treated with rehabilitation. More extensive brain damage may occur, leading to brain death or persistent vegetative state. Severe brain injury occurs in about two percent of patients who receive CPR. Patients who have extensive brain damage after resuscitation pose many ethical and legal questions.

DEFINITION OF DEATH

Brain death is a condition in which both the upper brain and the lower brain—or brain stem—have been destroyed.[3] In this case, body temperature, respiration, blood pressure, and hormones need to be artificially maintained in the intensive care unit.

No one has ever recovered from brain death. Brain-dead people can be maintained on a ventilator for days or months, and a brain-dead woman has been delivered of a live baby. Even if maximal medical support is used, though, all brain-dead people will eventually meet heart-lung death criteria also.

Brain death is legal death in most states. Patients who are brain dead do not have to be "withdrawn" from therapy. They are pronounced dead, and their ventilators or other systems are disconnected just as a ventilator is disconnected from a patient after an unsuccessful attempt at CPR. Brain death is not a matter of negotiation; it is an actual definition of death.

The concept of brain death is important for two practical reasons. First, it is unnecessary and irrational to maintain in intensive care a person who is legally dead. The cost of this "treatment" is tremendous. It would seem immoral to impoverish a deceased person's family or estate when further maintenance is absolutely futile. Again, we are referring only to brain-dead patients; patients in undefined coma, patients in PVS, and especially children with brain injury (whose ability to recover from coma is astounding) should be treated in an appropriate manner. But brain-dead patients are dead.

Second, patients who are brain dead are potential organ donors. Kidneys, corneas, and some other tissues (skin, bone) may be salvaged after heart-lung death, but hearts and livers deteriorate too quickly to be removed in these circumstances. The establishment of brain-death criteria enabled heart and liver transplantation and increased the success rate of many other organ transplants as well. Of course, patients (through signing their driver's license) or their families need to give consent before a brain-dead person's organs can be used for donation.

PEACE AND HOPE IN THE FACE OF DEATH

For the Christian, there is peace and hope in knowing that life does not cease with the last heartbeat or last brain wave. Mortal life is only one part of a larger reality, the eternal life that emanates from God and is possessed by believers through faith in Jesus Christ.

It is understandable that an unbeliever, who has no belief or hope in the eternal, may cling to the last thread of life. Actually, many believers are also frightened of death when actually faced with its grim reality. But when we link our lives with God by faith in Christ, we are no longer slaves to the fear of death (Hebrews 2:15). We are freed to fully live each day ordained for us, and we are released to allow death to be our doorway from this side to glory. Faith helps us as we seek guidance from the Word, pray for wisdom, and rest in God's grace.

The peace that comes through faith does not deny the painful reality of human grief, but if we know that the separation caused by death is only temporary (1 Thessalonians 4:13-18), we can find comfort and hope—and even joy—as we anticipate spending forever with the Lord and our loved ones. Knowing about Heaven can make it even more difficult to allow a family member who is not a believer to die, but in these cases we can still acknowledge that God's grace is beyond our understanding and control.

Jesus, when facing His own death, promised a sense of joy to His disciples: "You will grieve, but your grief will turn to joy" (John 16:20).

FOR DISCUSSION

Opening: Ask the group members to describe any experiences they or loved ones have had with terminal illness or CPR.

1. Jim, in conjunction with family members, his pastor, and Sally herself (pages 169-171), decided to discontinue Sally's intravenous fluids, thereby hastening her death rather than prolonging her struggle. As one of the participants in the decision, give your input.

2. Mrs. Hanson (pages 171-172) asked the doctor to pray that she would die.
   a. Individually, write out a brief prayer that you might use in this situation. Share your prayers as a group.
   b. Discuss how this approach is different from euthanasia.
   c. Is to pray in this way an expression of doubt that God will heal?

3. Eddie's parents signed a DNR order (page 175). Do you think they were justified in this? How were their attitudes as well as their own needs affected by the stress of the situation? If they had called you, as a friend, to help them make a decision, what would your advice be?

4. A surgeon must tell the family of a young child that exploratory surgery has confirmed the worst: terminal cancer with a prognosis of living just a few months. Using volunteers, role play the conversation in the waiting room before, during, and after the surgeon's visit. Use these characters: parent(s), sibling, pastor, uncle/aunt, surgeon. The surgeon's special assignment is to try to think of three ways to tell the truth about the cancer.

5. For three weeks, as a hospital nurse, you have been witnessing to Mr. Kaiser, an elderly man who is dying from prostate cancer. Just yesterday he seemed ready to make a decision for Christ, and today, as you visit, he seems open and ready to continue the conversation. Suddenly he collapses with cardiac arrest. Your first instinct is to call in the CPR team, but you hesitate for a moment because you know his chart has a DNR order plainly written on it, which you know expresses his own wishes. What do you do? How much is your decision linked to his spiritual state? Is it ethical to try to bring Mr. Kaiser back into a situation that may take him into excruciating pain, when now, if you let him go, he has avoided that? What will happen if you violate the DNR order?

NOTES:

1. Cicely Saunders and Edward Arnold, *The Management of Terminal Disease* (London: Hospital Medical Publishers, 1978).
2. David L. Schiedermayer, "The Decision to Forgo CPR in the Elderly Patient," *Journal of the American Medical Association*, October 14, 1988, 260:2096-2097.
3. President's Commission for the Study of Ethical Problems in Medicine and Biomedical and Behavioral Research, *Defining Death* (Washington, DC: U. S. Government Printing Office, 1981).

Chapter Eleven

Deciding Together

For Mary, the whole thing was like a nightmare. It seemed that she had only turned her back for an instant, just to answer the phone. But in that moment, three-year-old Suzie had squeezed through the fence and fallen into the pool.

Initially, there had been some hopeful signs. The emergency team had brought Suzie back with CPR. But now the doctors were saying that Suzie was brain dead and would never recover. Doctor Bunaphali had just suggested that Mary consider allowing transplant surgeons to remove Suzie's heart, liver, and kidneys for donation to other children.

Mary stood looking out the window of the ICU waiting room. On the busy street below, people rushed here and there, oblivious to her tragedy, helplessness, self-hatred, and remorse. Didn't anyone care that her little Suzie was dying? Did the doctor who was standing there care that she, herself, was dying inside? How can any mother decide to let someone cut out her daughter's heart, liver, and kidneys? Might the doctors be wrong about the diagnosis? She had never felt so alone.

Mary had moved to Los Angeles after a divorce, trying to start a new life for herself and Suzie. All she wanted was to give her little girl a new beginning. But they hadn't made any good friends yet, and they hadn't become involved in a church because Mary was afraid her divorce might be an issue.

She picked up the phone. "Mom," she started to cry. "Mom," she continued, after regaining some composure, "how can I tell you this? Suzie's been in an accident. She fell into the pool. They revived her, but she's on a lot of machines." Mary paused, listening to the barrage of questions mixed with incriminations. She had expected this; it was what had prevented her from calling earlier. She and her mother had never been close since her father had died. Along with the rest of her family, Mary's mother had blamed Mary for the divorce. Now they had another thing to blame her for.

Mary had been hoping for Suzie's miraculous recovery, so no one at home would ever need to know about this. But now she understood that it was too late. Breaking down completely, Mary handed the phone to the doctor. "Hello, Mrs. Ashley. My name is Doctor Bunaphali. Your daughter has been through a lot this week," he said, speaking slowly. "She has done very well, considering the circumstances, but now she may need some help deciding how to proceed. We are sure that Suzie will not recover and that her brain is now dead. We would like to suggest that the useful organs be removed before the respirator is disconnected. Is there anyone who can help Mary decide? We know this is a hard decision, but at least it would bring some good out of this tragedy."

Mary took the phone again. "Mom, I can't decide. Unplugging the machines seems just the same as killing her. But they tell me she is already dead anyway, in her brain. I just don't think I could live with the guilt. I need some help, Mom. I need somebody to hold me. This is too much to handle alone."

DECISIONS, DECISIONS

This book has been about issues and decisions, but most of all
it has been about peoples' lives and how we try to resolve the
dilemmas presented by common medical situations. Some of
the stories we've told have been based on our own personal
struggles with life-and-death decisions.

Ideally these decisions should be made together, with support from family, friends and church. Sadly, however, many
people face these paralyzing choices alone. Separated from
family, friends, and church support, Mary struggled to know
what was best. In the end, she agreed to the doctor's request.
But later she wondered, and for years she punished herself,
first of all for letting Suzie out of her sight and then for "giving
up hope," when maybe there was a one-in-a-million chance the
doctors were wrong and Suzie might have recovered. Perhaps a
miracle might have happened, she thought. Yet, she reasoned,
the decision wasn't about whether Suzie was dying—the doctor
said her brain was dead—but about whether or not to use her
organs to help other children.

When decisions like this arise for you, how will you decide?
Who will help you? Which principles will you use? What goals
or results will you have in mind? How will you move beyond
the potentially devastating residual loneliness, guilt, isolation,
and remorse?

Sometimes people say, "I can't decide." But of course not
to decide is to decide. And sometimes people say, "Doctor, you
decide." But to let the doctor decide is also to decide. And how
do you know on what basis he or she will proceed? One doctor,
when asked how he made decisions, said "I do what I would do
for my mother." But is his mother like yours? Is his relationship with his mother the same as your relationship with your
mother?

Important decisions incorporate our values and principles,
many of which are "caught" rather than taught. These principles affect our view of life and death and crucial concepts like

the meaning of faith, relationships, and honor.

What does it mean to honor our father and mother? What does it mean to respect the image of God in another human being? What does it mean to be human together in a world that includes inevitable pain, suffering, and loss, and which invariably brings events beyond our control? And after a decision has been reached, what does it mean for those who remain that God is forgiving and gracious?

BEYOND INDEPENDENCE AND ISOLATION

In recent years, changes in medicine and in society have influenced decision-making. For example, the development of *dialysis* brought difficult decisions about who should benefit from the new technology and who might forgo dialysis.[1]

Perhaps it seems that the problem is the new technology. "Life was simpler before," you might protest. "If people would just let nature take its course, we wouldn't be so bombarded and confused by these new issues." There is some merit in this argument. Common sense argues there must be some limits on our tampering with human reproduction. At the other end of the spectrum, that same common sense affirms that there is a time to die and that it is only vanity that motivates us to strive to resist death until the bitter end.

But technology is not the ultimate problem. It is also natural to die of measles, diphtheria, and polio. Would we really want to return to those days? Scientific discovery will bring ever more sophisticated methods to conquer disease, alleviate pain, postpone death, and assist in the creation of life. This creative drive to expand the horizons of knowledge is in general a good thing.

But power, whether it is the mighty power of a rushing river or the power to "create" and sustain life, can be directed and controlled. Uncontrolled, power can lead to disaster. In terms of medical ethics, direction and control come from within our culture: our values, our shared morality, our relatedness, our philosophy of life, our history. Normally these foundational factors shift gradually over time, but this century has seen rapid changes in our way of life—changes that influence the life-and-death decisions we've been considering.

Christy's Only Hope

Let's return to our story of Suzie and her mother, Mary.

At a different hospital in California, another three-year-old, Christy, desperately needs a new liver. She's been waiting for months, but has recently been hospitalized with terminal liver failure. Her prognosis is hopeless unless a transplant is done within a few days.

Christy's case has received national media attention. Her health maintenance organization (HMO) initially refused to cover the $100 thousand expense of the transplant on the basis that such therapy was specifically excluded in the contract.

So Christy's church got involved, and one of the members, a television commentator, made a public appeal for funds that raised, in less than a month, far more than the amount needed. In terms of values, there could be little doubt that the community still placed an extremely high value on the life of this particularly medically needy child.

A few politicians (though none were local) questioned spending this money for such a limited and uncertain end, when social justice (nationally and globally) required a more equitable distribution of resources. Others questioned the propriety of "going public" and the pressure this brought to bear on the allocation priority system of the National Organ Procurement and Transplantation Network.

Christy's parents and friends, however, were not at all concerned with statistics and uncertainties. Having raised the funds, their single focus now became the availability of a suitable donor before Christy died of liver failure.

Dr. Bunaphali knew of Christy's need when he talked to Suzie's mother, Mary. His own personal dilemma was how to remain objective, knowing that in all likelihood Suzie would never recover and that her liver could mean a new lease on life for Christy. Of course, he was not a transplant surgeon. And he never mentioned Christy's need to Mary, since this would have been undue pressure. In the end, Christy received Suzie's liver.

Mary wondered if she should have trusted Dr. Bunaphali. She had never requested a second opinion. She had assumed, instead, that Dr. Bunaphali spoke for the whole medical team and was concerned with Suzie's best interest.

Now, the more she thought about her daughter's death, the angrier she became, and her anger was intensified by her already intense feelings of remorse and sorrow. She began to wonder if she had any grounds for a malpractice suit against the hospital or Dr. Bunaphali.

The Importance of Relationships

The patient-doctor relationship has changed radically in just the past few years.[2] Until recently, the doctor was trusted to act as the patient's advocate, friend, and confidant, sometimes making decisions or pursuing treatment without the patient's knowledge or consent. Paternalism, or the attitude of "doctor knows best," was reflected by media programs in which (week after week) Dr. Kildare and Dr. Welby easily solved problems and healed diseases. People had an unrealistic perception of medicine and sometimes elevated physicians to divine status. And those in the medical field did little to discourage this image.

In recent years, a shift has occurred. The doctor-provider has become a purveyor of health services to the consumer-patient. The expenses are often paid by a third party that negotiates which therapies may or may not be covered. Doctors and patients feel financial pressures. Malpractice premiums may exceed $60 thousand. When a doctor needs to gross $100 thousand just to break even, it becomes harder to provide Marcus Welby-like care.

The threat of malpractice complicates the doctor's work

because it encourages excessive testing. "Defensive" medicine increases the risks to patients and increases the costs to the patient and to third-party payers. Also, defensive medicine creates an adversarial relationship between the doctor and patient.

Increasingly, patients are receiving care through corporate structures such as HMOs, with the result that a given patient must see a fixed group of doctors. HMO doctors are salaried employees, and this corporate arrangement can further complicate the doctor's ability to be a patient advocate.[3]

The net result of these factors is often mistrust and depersonalization. Technology has contributed to this distancing, often placing overt physical barriers—such as tubes, monitors, and a variety of sophisticated tests and hardware—between patient and doctor. A modern ICU seems to symbolize and even celebrate this dilemma. The triumph of medical technology can result in the dehumanization of the patient at the very time when the patient longs for a sense of human connectedness.

It is particularly ironic that medical science, which seeks to help people, can result in this kind of dehumanization. But of the many factors which have contributed to the changes we've been discussing, the lack of a spiritual view of human beings is perhaps the greatest problem. When man replaces God as the measure of all things, the system lacks a trustworthy standard.

If a human being can be reduced to only biochemical components, a mechanism that occasionally needs repair, is it any wonder that the doctor becomes a mere biomechanic? Then the consumer-patient who needs "fixing" contracts with the mechanic-provider to do the "repairs." When the results are less than perfect, the patient-doctor relationship is strained, and the result can be a malpractice lawsuit.

Another result of a man-centered philosophy of life is that as self becomes the primary concern, the self becomes the center around which all other realities must be organized. This is old-fashioned self-centeredness. The self then makes self-determination and sufficiency the most primal right. Quality of life then becomes the most decisive factor in the withdrawal of treatment. It is not surprising that these values have been displacing the sanctity of life as a primary principle in medical ethics, because the sanctity of life principle leads inexorably back to dependence on a Creator of life.

Self-sufficiency proudly proclaims disconnection: "Leave me alone." But life should not be that way.

A BETTER WAY TO MAKE DECISIONS

John Donne's view of life was very different than the modern man's. Writing in the early 1600s, he said,

> No man is an island unto himself; every man is a piece
> of the continent, a part of the main. If a clod be washed
> away by the sea, Europe is the less, as well as if a prom-
> ontory were, as well as if a manor of thy friend's or
> of thine own were: any man's death diminishes me,
> because I am involved in mankind, and therefore never
> send to know for whom the bell tolls; it tolls for thee.[4]

Donne was talking about community. With God as our Father, we are brothers and sisters, connected by faith and our experience as human beings made in His image. We are in this together.

If there is any single factor that modern Christians need to bring to life-and-death decisions, it is this: Christianity is a shared life. Christ shares His life with us, and we share it with each other. While in practice we may fall short of this ideal, shared life is a reality in the mind of God.

The sense of disconnection we often feel when facing decisions is one side effect of our modern context. But it is not only a modern feeling. The self-centered mind is not a twentieth-century invention. Recall Cain's protest: "Am I my brother's keeper?" (Genesis 4:9). For Christians, the answer is, "Yes. If my brother or sister needs me, I'll be there. We're in this together."

The most fundamental biblical moral imperative is the law of love. Fulfilling this imperative, as Christ did for us, means moving beyond an adolescent, self-centered focus to an inter-dependent community concern. We need each other. We are part of something which transcends disease or disability. We are part of the Body of Christ. We are part of something which transcends locality and space, time and culture. We are part of God's answer to the loneliness of grappling with life's issues. We are part of the community of believers, the family of God.

The Apostle Paul used the word *koinonia* to describe this connectedness, a Greek word often translated "fellowship," but which has a deeper meaning. In his letter to the Philippian church, Paul spoke of their participation (koinonia) in the gospel (1:5) and of their being all partakers of (koinonia) grace with him (1:7). In one of his most eloquent prayers, he prayed that their "love may abound more and more in knowledge and depth of insight, so that you may be able to discern what is best"(Philippians 1:9-11).

Surely these qualities would be helpful to someone facing a crucial decision in clinical ethics today. But is there not a certain sense in which such love, knowledge, and discernment are a corporate quality, a result of faith experienced together?

This brief epistle provides other principles that can be practically applied to medical-ethical decision-making. For example, as the apostle explains Christ's willingness to lay aside His rights in order to become a bond-servant for the good of man (Philippians 2:5-11), he exhorts the church:

Do nothing out of selfish ambition or vain conceit, but in humility consider others better than yourselves. Each of you should look not only to your own interests, but also to the interests of others. (Philippians 2:3-4)

Paul's is an attitude radically different from our self-centeredness. When we seek to serve others and give their best interests priority, ethical dilemmas in medicine emerge in a new light.

In chapter three of Philippians, Paul speaks of the surpassing value of knowing Christ. He explains that this special relationship includes the fellowship (koinonia) of Christ's sufferings, of being conformed to His death, of a process still being worked out even as he writes from his prison (3:1-14). Instead of seeking to escape the suffering that God had predicted (see Acts 9:16) and allowed, Paul embraces the suffering and becomes more like Christ.

If God is dead or simply disinterested and uninvolved, there is no place for this kind of thinking. Pain must be eradicated. Suffering is a problem to be eliminated. Persons who are suffering (from terminal illness, for example) or who might potentially suffer (such as severely handicapped newborns) can also be eliminated.

But our connectedness in Christ affirms God's purpose and His sovereignty. As Paul explains to a nonbelieving audience, "In him we live and move and have our being" (Acts 17:28). When the path He sets before us leads through the "fire," we know, along with Daniel's three friends (Daniel 3:25), that we never pass through the flames alone, for He is there with us, refining us into gold, as He did Job (Job 23:10).

Beyond this, when we affirm our shared life, we begin to understand that our suffering can be like a mirror in which we glimpse the eternal realities that escape us in good times. By rushing to eliminate pain and end suffering, we actually may be ignoring the grace and divine presence of God.

In our experience, we have found that with the support of others, persons can achieve their greatest work while dying: their greatest peace and their reconciliation with God, others, and themselves. In a sense, a person can become most integrated (whole) while disintegrating in a temporal sense. This is the "shalom" that Jesus gives, which surpasses all human comprehension and is able to guard both heart and mind (Philippians 4:6-7). Even after a decision is reached, when doubt and remorse can creep in, focusing our minds (together) on God's good things and practicing sincere faith bring a sense of the God of peace who is with us (Philippians 4:9).

However, such perspectives and results are not inevitable, even for sincere Christians. Death, dying, pain, and suffering are life's greatest challenges, regardless of the nature of one's faith. People who are experiencing severe stress need support. People facing life-and-death decisions need the corporate wisdom of the church. After the decision, and long after everyone else's life has returned to "normal," these brothers and sisters continue to need someone to help carry their burden. This fulfills the law of Christ (Galatians 6:2), for a burden shared is a burden lifted.

SOME WORDS OF ADVICE

A few thoughts might be helpful, especially for those actually facing crisis decisions in the realm of medical ethics:

1. If at all possible, do not make these decisions alone. You may not realize how deeply your perspective has been affected by pain and stress. If the decision involves yourself, your illness may affect your ability to sort out the conflicts and discern the best course. Just as a doctor should not treat himself, because his objectivity is impaired, a patient should try to avoid making decisions alone.[5]

2. Involve the church, difficult as it may be to ask for help. Ask for the elders (or other church leaders) as well as the pastor to become involved. If you desire, have them pray the "prayer of faith," which is really a combination of discernment coupled with confession of sins, supplication for healing, and acceptance of basic medical treatment—a truly whole-person approach (see James 5:13-16).

There is wisdom available to us when we ask God for it in faith (James 1:5), and there is "deliverance" in an abundance of counselors (Proverbs 11:14). One particular deliverance may be deliverance from self-doubt and remorse, which almost inevitably follow many of these decisions. Having prayerfully sought the Lord's guidance with a group of believers, once a decision has been reached and a direction taken, the responsibility for the results is also a shared experience.

3. In relation to medical advice, it is always acceptable to gather as much information as possible. Patients and families should ask their doctors, attend classes, watch programs, and read books about their illnesses. Patients and families may wish to join support groups which can provide credible and easy-to-understand information about certain diseases. They should request a second opinion and specialty consultation to gather more information when appropriate. Especially when there is medical uncertainty or a crucial life or death decision to be made, additional sources of factual input can be very helpful. Sometimes people under stress find it difficult to suggest additional input into their case, for fear that their primary doctor will be offended. But caring physicians want to know as much as possible about their patient's case and should be receptive to a second opinion.

4. In addition to factual information and medical opinion, it is also appropriate to seek ethical opinion. An increasing number of hospitals have ethics committees or ethics consultants available to assist patients and families as they confront decisions.

5. Prepare your mind in advance, if possible—especially in terms of the biblical texts, concepts, and principles that will guide your decisions. Expect conflict instead of easy answers. But remember that while some alternatives acceptable to the secular mind may not be acceptable to the Christian mind, most Christian alternatives will fall within acceptable secular parameters.

6. Try to have realistic expectations. While medicine utilizes science, it is basically an art. Actually, it is a ministry, which many doctors, especially some Christian doctors, under-

stand. Not everything that is broken can be fixed. Not everyone who is sick can be healed. Shared decision-making is essential. The integrity of the patient-doctor relationship, which is a major factor in life-and-death decisions, will best be maintained if the general approach is one of mutual trust. Truly, we (doctor and patient) must work together in this effort to discern the right thing to do, and to do the very best we can.

FOR DISCUSSION

Opening: Have each group member describe one difficult ethical decision in medicine he or she made. Was the decision made alone, as a part of a family group, or including other resource persons? If they had that decision to make again, what would they decide differently?

1. At your invitation, your neighbor Mary (pages 181-183) has become a member of your prayer group. It is one year after Suzie's death. You were amazed to discover how isolated Mary was as she grappled with this tragedy, and you wish you had been more sensitive to her needs. You are also amazed at the depth of her continuing pain—she seems to relive the experience daily. She brings it up every week to the group, and now she has begun calling group members daily to ask advice about whether she should file a malpractice suit.

   As a group, role-play what might be a typical weekly meeting. Have one person be Mary, one the friend who invited her, and the rest the ones who have been receiving calls from her lately.

2. Discuss the value of having a Christian doctor, both for treatment and for help in decision-making. List characteristics that would make a difference to you personally. Which is more important—medical expertise, compassion, or Christian profession?

3. The "law of love" is the consistent foundation of God's moral imperative for His people. The Old Testament directives to love God and our neighbor as ourselves (Leviticus 19:18) were reinforced by Jesus: "All the Law and the Prophets hang on these two commandments" (Matthew 22:34-40). In His life and teachings, we see many examples of loving and caring that can guide our decision-making in medical ethics. Have someone read each of the following texts, pausing after each reading to discuss as a group what principle(s) or examples might apply to life-and-death decisions:

   a. Matthew 7:12, The Golden Rule
   b. Matthew 8:1-4, A Leper Cleansed
   c. Matthew 25:31-40, The Sheep and the Goats
   d. Mark 3:31-35, Jesus' Mother and Brothers
   e. Mark 7:9-13, Honor Your Father and Mother
   f. Luke 18:15-17, The Kingdom Belongs to Little Children
   g. John 15:13, No Greater Love Than This

4. As Jesus touched people, bringing a sense of connection into their isolation and despair, so the church continues to have the duty and privilege to touch the hurting. In John 15, Jesus speaks of this shared life figuratively: He is the vine, and we are the branches. Paul uses the human body to speak of the same reality. Read 1 Corinthians 12:12-26 and discuss how the church might become more effective in supporting people in a medical ethics crisis, both before and after their decision.

5. Many doctors observe that the closer we get to death, the more we cling to life. In other words, while people in good health may say they would rather die than be maintained on life supports, when they become terminally ill they usually prefer to live on than die.

   a. Why do you think this may be true?
   b. Describe your own perspectives on death and dying.
   c. How does personal faith affect the way we die?

APPENDIX: A CHECKLIST FOR MAKING DECISIONS

Gather Information
___ Diagnosis
___ Treatment options
___ Benefits versus risks (including side effects)
___ Treatment recommendation of attending physician
___ Additional medical consultation(s)
___ Prognosis (likely outcome)
___ Costs and resources
___ Time frame for reaching decision (urgency)

Consider Factors
___ Patient's wishes (including advance directives such as Living Will or Durable Power of Attorney)
___ Expectations of patient and/or family
___ Patient's relationship to God
___ Patient's reconciliations with family/friends
___ Costs and resources

List Principles Involved
___ Principles of medical ethics
___ Principles of biblical ethics
___ Specific biblical texts

Acceptable Options/Directions
___ Acceptable by secular standards
___ Acceptable by biblical standards
___ Acceptable to patient/surrogate
___ Acceptable to family
___ Acceptable to church support system

Utilize Resources
___ Medical consultant
___ Ethics committee or consultant

___ Family support (emotional/spiritual/discernment/
economic)
___ Spiritual (pastor/church)
___ Social services
___ Psychological
___ Financial
___ Other agencies, such as hospice

Make Decision—Prayerfully

Commit your way unto the Lord. Let the peace of Christ
stand guard over your heart and mind. Remember that we
live always in the realm of the grace of God.

NOTES:
1. Steven Neu and Carl M. Kjellstrand, "Stopping Long-Term Dialysis: An
Empirical Study of Withdrawal of Life-Supporting Treatment," *New England
Journal of Medicine*, January 2, 1986, 314:14-20.
2. Mark Siegler, "The Progression of Medicine: From Physician Paternalism to
Patient Autonomy to Bureaucratic Parsimony," *Archives of Internal Medicine*,
April 1985, 145:713-715.
3. Frederick R. Abrams, "Patient Advocate or Secret Agent," *Journal of the
American Medical Association*, October 3, 1986, 256:1784-1785.
4. Erwin P. Rudolph, ed., *The John Donne Treasury* (Wheaton, IL: Victor Books,
1978), p. 34.
5. Alan Stoudemire and John M. Rhoads, "When the Doctor Needs a Doctor:
Special Considerations for the Physician-Patient," *Annals of Internal Medicine*, May 1983, pp. 654-659.

Glossary

ALZHEIMER'S DISEASE. One of several types of DEMENTIA. A degenerative disease of unknown cause that begins with memory loss and may progress to severe disability and nearly complete loss of higher brain function.

AMNIOCENTESIS. An obstetrical procedure whereby a needle is inserted through the mother's abdominal wall into the uterus to remove some of the amniotic fluid in which the baby is floating; this fluid can be analyzed in an effort to determine if the baby is suffering from certain chemical or genetic defects.

ARTIFICIAL INSEMINATION. Installation of sperm into the vagina or uterus by medical technique rather than by intercourse. If the husband's sperm is used, it is called AIH (artificial insemination, homologous). If donor sperm is used, it is called AID (artificial insemination, donor).

CARDIOPULMONARY RESUSCITATION (CPR). The emergency medical technique used to try to revive someone when their heart stops beating or they stop breathing.

CONGENITAL. Present at birth.

CONSANGUINITY. Pertaining to the offspring of two closely related people.

CORTICAL. Referring to the cerebral cortex, that part of the brain where higher functions occur (i.e., memory, speech, voluntary movement, sensation).

DEBILITATION. A state of marked weakness or infirmity.

DEMENTIA. The condition of deteriorated mental function that may occur with ALZHEIMER'S DISEASE, brain injury, or many other causes. (Also defined in chapter 7, appendix.)

DIALYSIS. The process of filtering and cleansing the blood using an artificial kidney when a person's kidneys no longer work.

DOWN SYNDROME. A combination of genetically determined birth defects (previously known as Mongolism) that includes varying degrees of mental retardation and characteristic structural anomalies.

ECHOCARDIOGRAM. A way of producing a picture of the heart using ultrasound waves instead of x-rays. It helps in determining the structure and function of the heart.

ELECTROENCEPHALOGRAM (EEG). The electrical recording of brain waves.

EMBRYO. The earliest stage of development of an organism. In human development, the embryo stage lasts from fertilization through six weeks. The early embryonic stage can be subdivided (ZYGOTE, morula, blastocyst, etc.), and the late embryonic stage merges into the fetal stage. All these names are attempts to describe a continuous process.

ESOPHAGUS. That part of the upper gastro-intestinal tract that carries swallowed food from the mouth to the stomach.

EUGENICS. The philosophy and science that attempts to improve the hereditary qualities of a race (or breed). Methods include control of mating, selective sterilization, and selective abortion.

FALLOPIAN TUBE. The earthworm-sized tubes attached to both sides of the uterus. The outer end is open and actively captures eggs released from the ovary at the time of ovulation.

FEEDING TUBE. *See* TUBE FEEDING.

GAMETE. Reproductive cells. Eggs and sperm are both gametes.

GESTATIONAL. Having to do with pregnancy.

HEMOPHILIA. A hereditary disease (that affects only males) in which the blood lacks sufficient amounts of a chemical for normal clotting. People with hemophilia are prone to internal or external hemorrhage with injury, and require injection of the missing blood factor, which is obtained from serum from people without the disease.

HOSPICE. A concept of care for people who are terminally ill.

It attempts to meet the medical, emotional, social, and spiritual needs of the patient and his or her family.

IMAGO DEI. Based on Genesis 1:26, this Latin phrase means "image of God," a crucial concept in anyone's view of personhood or the value of human life. If God made us, somehow, like Himself, and all human beings are therefore bearers of His image, life is sacred. Our rather basic explanation is that this concept speaks of spiritual realities (as opposed to thinking that human beings, for instance, physically resemble God). In saying this, however, we would not want to deny the biblical perspective on the importance of body as well as soul/spirit when we think of man in a truly wholistic sense.

IN-VITRO FERTILIZATION (IVF). A technique whereby a woman's egg is taken from her body and placed in a culture dish to which sperm are added. When fertilization has occurred, the embryo is placed in the woman's uterus, where it develops as any normal pregnancy.

IRRADIATION. Exposing a cancer patient to radioactive radiation so that the cancer cells will hopefully die faster than normal cells. It occasionally cures the cancer, but it is more often used to slow the cancer growth.

ISOLETTE. An "incubator" that allows a newborn to be kept at a constant temperature, given extra oxygen, and be monitored and observed closely.

LAPAROSCOPY. A surgical procedure that allows the surgeon to look at the pelvic organs and/or perform minor surgical procedures through a small telescope that is inserted through a small incision in the abdominal wall.

MENINGITIS. An infection of the tissue that covers the brain.

When caused by viruses, it usually resolves without after-effects. When caused by bacteria, it is fatal unless treated quickly and aggressively.

NEONATAL. Refers to the newborn period. Neonatology is a subspecialty of pediatrics that cares for newborns.

OVULATION. The release of one or more eggs by an ovary.

PERSISTENT VEGETATIVE STATE (PVS). A condition in which the upper part of the brain is severely damaged so that the person is unable to think, feel, or do; but the lower part of the brain, which controls vital functions like breathing, is still able to function. Karen Anne Quinlan was in PVS.

PREEMIE. A premature newborn.

PROGNOSIS. Outlook; prediction for the future, based on experience with similar cases.

PROSTAGLANDIN. A hormone that has many physiological effects, including the ability to cause the uterus to contract in labor even in early pregnancy.

SONOGRAPHY. An imaging technique that produces pictures of internal organs using sound waves instead of x-rays; used commonly in obstetrics to monitor the size and structure of the unborn baby.

SPINA BIFIDA. A birth defect that involves a cleft of part of the bones of the spine, allowing a protrusion of the membranes that cover the spinal cord; the spinal cord and nerves may be involved; neurological deficit may be negligible or severe.

SURROGATE. Someone appointed to act in place of another.

TUBE FEEDING. An artificial means of feeding for people unable to swallow; a soft, flexible tube is inserted into the stomach through the mouth, the nose, or surgically through the abdominal wall.

UTILITARIANISM. The school of ethical thought that strives for the greatest good for the greatest number of people; often capsulized as "the end justifies the means."

VIABLE. Capable of survival. In relation to obstetrics, it refers to the ability of the baby to live outside the uterus when it is sufficiently mature.

X AND Y SPERM ISOLATION. Separation of sperm from a semen sample into those that will produce male (Y) offspring and those that will produce female (X) offspring. It is a method of sex selection. (Sperm, not eggs, determine the sex of a baby.)

ZYGOTE. The EMBRYO stage of development is divided into several shorter stages. The first is the zygote, which is from conception until the fertilized egg has divided into four cells.

Suggestions for Further Reading

CHAPTER 1—MEDICAL ETHICS

Beauchamp, Tom L., and James F. Childress. *Principles of Biomedical Ethics*. 3rd ed. New York: Oxford University Press, 1989.

Excellent discussion of the various principles and theories of ethics.

Jonsen, Albert R., Mark Siegler, and W.J. Winslade. *Clinical Ethics: A Practical Approach to Ethical Decisions in Clinical Medicine*. 2nd ed. New York: Macmillan, 1986.

Short, readable discussion of clinical ethics. Case studies of informed consent, treatment refusal, do-not-resuscitate orders, etc., make this an important and practical book.

Kass, Leon R. *Toward a More Natural Science: Biology and Human Affairs*. New York: The Free Press, 1985.

Kass is concerned about the doctor-patient relationship; his thoughtful analysis of the meaning of the Hippocratic Oath is the best anywhere.

Lammers, Stephen E., and Allen Verhey. *On Moral Medicine: Theological Perspectives in Medical Ethics*. Grand Rapids, MI: Eerdmans, 1987.

A wide-ranging collection of ethics codes and essays from authors as diverse as C. S. Lewis and Ivan Illich. A good reference volume.

Siegler, Mark, P.A. Singer, and David L. Schiedermayer. *Medical Ethics: An Annotated Bibliography*. Philadelphia: American College of Physicians, 1989.

A short, annotated bibliography emphasizing recent and important papers on ethics that appeared in high-impact medical journals or featured empirical data collection.

CHAPTER 2—MAKING SARAH LAUGH

McIlhaney, Joe S., and S. Nethery. *1250 Health-Care Questions Women Ask With Straightforward Answers by an Obstetrician/Gynecologist*. Grand Rapids, MI: Baker Book House, 1985.

This book provides practical answers for women about their health from a Christian specialist in gynecology.

Schiedermayer, David L. "May the Lord Judge Between Us." *Christian Medical Society Journal*. Summer 1988, XIX(2).

A discussion of surrogate motherhood and the ethics of the new reproductive technologies with reference to the Old Testament.

CHAPTER 3—MOMMY'S RIGHTS, BABY'S RIGHTS

Perkins, S. "The Pro-Life Credibility Gap." *Christianity Today.*
April 21, 1989.
      This is a call by a black evangelical pastor for pro-
lifers to look beyond the issue of abortion to a commitment
to the lives they save.

Shettles, L., and D. Rorvik. *Rites of Life.* Grand Rapids, MI:
Zondervan, 1983.
      A readable and accurate description of embryological
development followed by discussion of the relevance of
this information in the abortion debate.

Sider, Ronald J. *Completely Pro-Life.* Downers Grove, IL: Inter-
Varsity Press, 1987.
      The executive director of Evangelicals for Social Action
tries to expand the vision of pro-life individuals from one-
issue thinking and activism to a broader Christian understanding of justice.

Stafford, Tim. "The Abortion Wars." *Christianity Today.* October 6, 1989.
      A brief look at the opposition to abortion that has
surfaced during three periods in the past two thousand
years.

Waltke, Bruce K. "Reflections from the Old Testament on Abortion." *Christian Medical Society Journal.* Vol. XIX, No. 1.
Winter/Spring, 1988.
      This is a scholarly look at humaneness and the nature
of the fetus from the words of the Old Testament.

CHAPTER 4—THE DREADED SURPRISE

Deciding to Forgo Life-Sustaining Treatment. The President's
Commission. U.S. Government Printing Office, 1983.

Chapter 6 of this comprehensive report looks at the medical, ethical, and public policy issues of seriously ill newborns.

Horan, D.J., and M. Delahoyde, eds. *Infanticide and the Handicapped Newborn.* Provo, UT: Brigham Young University, 1982.
This well-referenced collection of essays by noted writers from medicine, law, and philosophy is a strong defense of the imperiled newborn.

Schaeffer, Francis A., and C. Everett Koop. *Whatever Happened to the Human Race?* Old Tappan, NJ: Revell, 1979.
An evangelical theologian and pediatric surgeon give a thorough pro-life discussion of abortion, infanticide, and euthanasia.

CHAPTER 5—WHAT WOULD JOHN WANT?

Culver, Charles M., and Bernard Gert. *Philosophy in Medicine.* New York: Oxford University Press, 1982.
This discussion of the philosophical underpinnings of the practice of medicine is unusually clear and straightforward. Chapter three, on valid consent and competence, is exceptional.

Katz, Jay. *The Silent World of Doctor and Patient.* New York: The Free Press, 1984.
An eye-opening look at the doctor-patient decision-making process.

Ramsey, Paul. *The Patient as Person.* Yale University Press, 1970.
This book looks at birth, death, illness, and injury as events in human lives and specifically addresses several

current problems in medical ethics. Chapter one is a person-centered discussion of consent.

CHAPTER 6—THE PLAGUE

Christianity Today. August 7, 1987.
   The focus of this entire issue is on Christian attitudes toward AIDS and persons with AIDS. Several perspectives are offered.

Koop, C. Everett. "Physician Leadership in Preventing AIDS." *Journal of the American Medical Association,* 1987; 258:2111.
   The Surgeon General argues persuasively that physicians must play a key leadership role in preventing the further spread of AIDS.

Shilts, Randy. *And the Band Played on: Politics, People, and the AIDS Epidemic.* New York: St. Martin's Press, 1987.
   Shilts, a San Francisco newspaper reporter, traces the political and scientific response to AIDS during the early years of the epidemic. He also gives an account of patient Zero, a promiscuous homosexual flight attendant who is thought to have transmitted the virus to numerous men in multiple cities.

CHAPTER 7—THE FINAL YEARS

Gillies, John. *A Guide to Caring for & Coping With Aging Parents.* Nashville: Thomas Nelson Publishers, 1981.
   A practical guidebook written from the author's own experiences, giving useful information from a Christian perspective.

Mace, Nancy L., and Peter V. Robins P. *The 36-Hour Day: A Family Guide to Caring for Persons with Alzheimer's Disease, Related Dementing Illnesses and Memory Loss Later*

in Life. Johns Hopkins University Press, 1981.
    An insightful and helpful guide to dealing with the realities of Alzheimer's disease.

CHAPTER 8—A NON-TREATMENT OF CHOICE

Lynn, Joanne, ed. *By No Extraordinary Means: The Choice to Forgo Life-Sustaining Food and Water.* Indiana University Press, 1986.
    Twenty-seven authors from many disciplines contribute their current perspectives and insights regarding the use of artificial fluids and nutrition.

CHAPTER 9—*MERCY* KILLING?

Hastings Center Report. Vol. 19, No. 1. January/February 1989.
    This special supplement has nine articles that give a variety of perspectives on euthanasia.

Horan, Dennis J., and David Mall, eds. *Death, Dying and Euthanasia.* Washington, DC: University Publications of America, 1977.
    This is an excellent collection of short writings by some of the best thinkers. It presents ethical, religious, legal, and medical perspectives.

CHAPTER 10—WHEN IT'S ONLY A MATTER OF TIME

Richards, Lawrence O., and Paul Johnson. *Death & the Caring Community.* Portland, OR: Multnomah Press, 1980.
    From Multnomah's Critical Concern Series, this book is about ministering to the terminally ill with a message of hope and eternal life.